INNOVATIONS IN HELPING CHRONIC PATIENTS

COLLEGE STUDENTS IN A MENTAL INSTITUTION

INNOVATIONS IN HELPING CHRONIC PATIENTS

COLLEGE STUDENTS IN A MENTAL INSTITUTION

Julian Rappaport
Department of Psychology
University of Illinois
Urbana-Champaign, Illinois

Jack M. Chinsky
Department of Psychology
University of Connecticut
Storrs, Connecticut

Emory L. Cowen
Department of Psychology
University of Rochester
Rochester, New York

ACADEMIC PRESS New York and London 1971

ACADEMIC PRESS, INC.
111 Fifth Avenue, New York, New York 10003

United Kingdom Edition published by
ACADEMIC PRESS, INC. (LONDON) LTD.
24/28 Oval Road, London NW1 7DD

Library of Congress Catalog Card Number: 72-182557

PRINTED IN THE UNITED STATES OF AMERICA

CONTENTS

Preface vii
Acknowledgments xi

Chapter 1. **The Issues and the Problems**
I. Treatment of Profound Psychological Disorder 1
II. Manpower Considerations 9
III. New Manpower Utilizations in the Mental Hospital 12
IV. The Effectiveness of Nonprofessionals 22
V. Helper Attributes 28
VI. Summary and Overview 35

Chapter 2. **The State Hospital: A Sleeping Dragon**
I. The Mental Hospital 37
II. The Pilot Project: The Dragon Stirring 45
III. Changing the University's Social System 49

Chapter 3. **An Overview**
I. Design of the Study 57
II. Evaluation 59
III. Major Questions and Findings 61

Chapter 4. **Patients, Process, and Students**
I. Patients and Patient Evaluation 64
II. Meetings and Process Evaluation 74
III. Students 78

Chapter 5. **Research Evaluation: Patients**

I.	Attendance and Process Data	85
II.	Pretest Data	87
III.	Major Outcome Evaluations	91
IV.	Relationship between Patient Characteristics and Change Scores	102
V.	Patient Perceptions of the College Students	106
VI.	Follow-Up Study	110
VII.	Some General Observations	111
VIII.	Summary	113

Chapter 6. **Research Evaluation: College Students**

I.	Student Personality and Patient Outcome	114
II.	Student Leaders versus Nonvolunteer Controls: Personality Measures	126
III.	Student Leaders versus Nonvolunteer Controls: Initial Attitudes and Attitude Change	128
IV.	Group Process Measures	133

Chapter 7. **The Project from a Human Perspective**

I.	Introduction	138
II.	The "Tune-Up" Period	139
III.	Initiation Day	140
IV.	Finding the Meeting Rooms	142
V.	Scheduling the Meetings	143
VI.	Student Reactions	145
VII.	The Hospital Staff	147
VIII.	The Patients	149
IX.	The First Meeting	149
X.	Patient Group Meetings	154
XI.	The "Special" Group	166
XII.	Termination	167
XIII.	Farewell	169
XIV.	Student and Hospital Reactions to Outcome	170
XV.	Follow-Up Interview with Students	171

Chapter 8. **Concluding Observations**

I.	The Patients	182
II.	Lessons Learned and To Be Learned	184
III.	Future Prospects	185
IV.	Student Volunteers	186
V.	The Setting	188
VI.	Summing Up	188

References 190

Index 199

PREFACE

This volume at its deepest roots was stimulated by a fundamental principle of the community mental health and community psychology movement: "the helper–therapy principle." In the process of reaching out to those with problems in living, the "helper" may help himself. This principle has been seen to operate with indigenous nonprofessionals—those from within the ranks of the target group. In the present work the helpers are not indigenous to the target group. On the surface, college students and chronic patients have little in common. Yet, in important psychosocial ways they share similar problems: Chronic patients are alienated from the larger society, they are "marginal men"; in many ways so too are college students. Perhaps never before has a group with such a vast reservoir of energy and potential been so untapped by a society. One result of this failure to utilize resources, i.e., through not hearing students' demands for "relevance" and a meaningful voice in altering their own environment, is the frequently noted indifference, apathy, and frustration of many college students. What this volume attempts to examine is the extent to which these very real student needs can be channeled into constructive social action. Our view was that students' enthusiasm for social and humanitarian change could be mobilized to have a positive impact on a hospital and its residents, as well as on the students themselves.

Thus, in significant ways the project described in this volume is both a tertiary prevention program for chronic hospitalized patients and a primary prevention program for students. The patient-rehabilitative goals of the program are obvious. More subtle, and consequently more difficult to evaluate, is its primary preventive potential. The use of college students in helping and social change roles may both enable them to deal constructively with societal problems, and to understand the problems of community health. Regardless of their later career decisions, participation in a live, human-service helping program should facilitate development of a deeper understanding of psychological problems, which would be helpful in their own education of family, friends, and neighbors.

This book considers only one of many roles that college students can play in the pursuit of social relevance. All three authors continue to work with college students in a variety of human-service roles and settings. The latter range from elementary, junior high, and high schools, to ghetto homes, settlement houses, courts, clinics, and hospitals. Each setting has its own set of goals and problems, and each has its own double-edged intention of facilitating the growth of identified target groups and participating students.

This vital component of the project has been extended not only to other social problems but to numerous nonprofessional caregivers as well. Programs using a variety of nontraditional mental health workers (e.g., housewives, indigenous neighborhood youth, retired oldsters, high-school students, elementary-school students) have been successfully linked with a number of groups requiring help (e.g., nursery- and elementary-school children, pregnant mothers) to mutual advantage. The need for such programs continues to grow not only because we lack sufficient manpower to conquer social ills but also because increasing numbers of individuals are available for meaningful, socially constructive activities. The four-day work week is almost a reality. As leisure time increases, many more people will have time to devote to other than survival concerns. The currently evident dilemma of the alienated, apathetic college student with considerable human-service potential but no outlet, could well be repeated on a much wider and more devastating scale in our society. In addition to examining carefully those social forces operating to increase recreation and retirement time, we need also to legitimize, and provide mechanisms for, increasing numbers of people to become involved in social service activities. Hopefully, the material in this book, demonstrating benefit to both the helper and helped, will serve to model this needed emphasis.

This book is specifically written for researchers, students, professional and nonprofessional caregivers. In addition to program description and analysis, the volume presents a detailed report of the outcome of a project using college students as mental health workers. Included is a comprehensive research report evaluating the program's impact on both patients and students. Suggestions for future selection, training, and programming are also included.

In addition to its research perspective, the volume deals with three focal issues. First is the problem of institutional innovation. The volume heavily emphasizes our efforts to mobilize an entrenched custodial institution to develop active treatment programs. Second, the volume is concerned with treatment for chronic hospitalized mental patients, considered by the Joint Commission on Mental Health and Illness to be the core problem and unfinished business of the mental health movement. Finally, we describe an attempt to involve college students in relevant roles designed to reduce problems of perceived irrelevant education and alienation. The latter portion of the book describes specific experiences and reactions of college students in a mental hospital; as such, it may serve as a vicarious journey for others contemplating such an experience.

ACKNOWLEDGMENTS

A project the size and length of this one, spanning four years from conception to completion, and involving almost 400 different people, inevitably depends on more than a few individuals for success. This study could not have been undertaken without the many hours of time so generously given to it by Dr. Thomas Irwin, Chief Psychologist at the Rochester State Hospital. Special gratitude is also due the college students whose participation in the seminar and practicum experiences taught the authors far more than we could have taught them. To the more than 320 patients who participated in this project, appreciation is extended in the hope that it may have made their own lives, in some small way, more meaningful.

Although Rochester State Hospital is, of course, the focus of this study, it should be clear that the need for institutional reform extends to almost every state mental hospital in the country. Moreover, by highlighting those aspects of the hospital situation that need reform, we have neglected to mention the many positive features of Rochester State. The authors are indebted to Dr. Guy Walters, Rochester State's former Superintendent, Miss Ruth Lewis, Chief of Nurses, and to the many hospital staff members who aided us in this project.

The research was partially supported by the Department of Psychology of the University of Rochester, and by the Maurice Falk Medical Fund, Pittsburgh, Pennsylvania. Additional support was obtained from grant number 0215-35-122 of the University of Connecticut Research Foundation. Portions of the manuscript were completed while the first author was a University of Illinois Summer Faculty Fellow, and while the second author was supported by a University of

Connecticut Summer Research Fellowship. Portions of the research were done with the support of the National Science Foundation (grant number GJ-9) and the National Institute of Mental Health.

A grant for materials used in student–patient groups was given to the project by the Alpha Phi Omega service fraternity of the University of Rochester.

Many other individuals played important roles in the completion of the tasks of this project. Those who deserve special mention include Professors Edward Ware and Michael Davidson who were invaluable statistical consultants. Other faculty members at the University of Rochester who helped on the project were Drs. Melvin Zax, Harotun Babigian, and Vincent Nowlis. Thanks are also extended to Dr. Paul Goldring who helped to teach the seminar, and to Joan Huser Liem and Morton Saloman whose consultation to both the authors and the college students was of great value. Arlene Rappaport was responsible for the art work necessary for the completion of the Figure–Ground Confusion Test. Much of the clerical and computational work was completed by Mary Hartshorn and Carolyn Norris. Typing at various stages of illegible writing was completed by Mrs. Linda Kibby and Mrs. Dorothy DeMotte.

Finally, the authors wish to thank their wives, Arlene, Vivian, and Renee whose emotional support and understanding were a major component of their ability to complete the many tasks involved in producing this volume.

Chapter 1

THE ISSUES AND THE PROBLEMS

Two of the most challenging problems facing the mental health fields today are the ineffectiveness of treatment approaches for profound, chronic psychological dysfunction and critical professional manpower shortages. The work described in this volume probes the extent to which convergent, mutually supportive resolutions can be brought to bear on these problems. A central question that has engaged us is how effective are relatively naive, untrained college students as helping agents with chrònic mental hospital patients. Before considering the specifics of the investigation, however, it is appropriate to explore the underlying considerations that motivate it.

I. TREATMENT OF PROFOUND PSYCHOLOGICAL DISORDER

A. A Brief History of Our Progress

Historically, man's earliest concern with disordered behavior was restricted to extreme deviance and to the highly bizarre. Concerted efforts to cope with such conditions can be traced back well over 2000 years (Zax & Cowen, 1972). Initially, only when behavior went seriously awry and threatened others did it attract attention. Viewed over a span of 20 centuries, it is apparent that expansion of the definitional scope of abnormal psychology has been an infinitesimally slow process, only occasionally accelerated by more dramatic events. Only gradually have we come to accept the multifaceted, sometimes subtle and indirect, ways in which psychological problems gain expression, and how emotional dysfunction is intimately intertwined with other conditions of living. For example, we now include conditions such as character defects, psychosomatic disorders, and philosophical and existential neuroses within the domain of the mental health specialist. In prior years, such conditions would either have been handled by another specialist, such as a physician or clergyman, or would have gone unrecognized as psychological problems. Indeed, broadening of scope is such that today many are willing to consider as a legitimate activity the involvement of mental health professionals in tasks such as job training or social-political action (O'Connor & Rappaport, 1970).

Even with these obvious and significant expansions in focus, society's greatest efforts have always been invested in the most puzzling of all psychological disorders—the functional psychoses. Even today, broad sections of modern society and many primitive ones still recognize only highly deviant, florid, indisputable departures from reality as causes for genuine concern.

Thus, while society's views about the nature of disordered psychological behavior have broadened, an unswerving conviction has remained that the greatest challenge to the mental health fields is that of evident and profound dysfunction. When, a decade ago, the Joint Commission on Mental Illness and Health was established "to analyze and evaluate the needs and resources of the mentally ill in the United States and to make recommendations for a national mental health program (Joint Commission Report, 1961, p. vii)," its most central conclusion and recommendation was as follows: "A national mental health program should recognize that major mental illness is the core problem and unfinished business of the mental health movement, and that intensive treatment of patients with critical and prolonged mental breakdowns should have first call on fully trained members of the mental health professions [p. 14]." Although serious questions have been raised at the conceptual level about the wisdom of allocating the lion's share of sharply limited mental health resources to treatment of the profoundly ill (Cowen & Zax, 1967; Zax & Cowen, 1972), the preceding statement clearly reflects the dominant place and central challenge of major mental illness in the hierarchy of concerns of responsible mental health professionals. As Braginsky, Braginsky, and Ring (1969, p. 27) put it: "Other than war itself, there is perhaps no human problem of such manifest significance that has remained so elusive as mental illness."

Given the widespread recognition accorded to the challenge of major mental illness, particularly schizophrenia, and given man's intensive effort to cope with such conditions, it is important that we carefully examine our cumulative record of success in this area.

Scheff (1966) indicates that more than 5000 studies on the etiology and treatment of schizophrenia alone were reported in the literature between 1920 and 1965. These studies embrace a broad spectrum of theories of causation and a wide variety of treatment approaches. Yet, he concludes that these, as well as countless preceding contributions spanning centuries, have failed completely to resolve basic issues of cause and cure in the functional psychoses. Similarly, intensive reviews of more delimited segments of this broad area such as those emphasizing organic factors (Arieti, 1955) or biochemical factors (Kety, 1967) pessimistically conclude that causative agents or effective treatment procedures within each of these subdomains remain as yet unidentified. Other writers have gone a step further in suggesting that much of what has been done so far has not only failed to advance treatment but has actually impeded it (Braginsky *et al.*, 1969). A recent, extensive review of the literature (Paul, 1969) underscores the conclusion that, once rooted and established, mental illness is highly resistant to fundamental, enduring correction. That our record in this area is thus far so dismal is due far less to lack of interest, imaginativeness or dedication and far more to the totally baffling, refractory nature of the disorders themselves.

Past failures, rather than discouraging investigators, have seemingly stimulated even more intensive study. The breadth of current exploration is extraordinary, ranging from environmental-preventive approaches, on the one side, to genetic and biochemical approaches, on the other. This breadth is clearly illustrated in a recent volume on the origins of schizophrenia, (Romano, 1967b) that reflects some of the most advanced current thinking and work in this area, none of which as yet gives promise of approaching a major breakthrough. Similarly, while Paul (1969) singles out the milieu and behavior modification approaches to chronic mental illness as prospectively worthwhile, he is far from suggesting that we are on the threshold of a basic solution to this pressing social problem.

B. Treatment Approaches with Psychotic Patients

Our thesis to this point is summarized simply by the contention that the history of society's efforts to cope with profound psychological dysfunction has been one of overwhelming failure. Although few would contest the accuracy of that statement, it does not describe the ways in which treatment of the psychotic has been approached and the reasons motivating such approaches. These issues have been extensively considered elsewhere (Selling, 1940; Zilboorg & Henry, 1941; Alexander & Selesnick, 1966; Zax & Cowen, 1972). From these accounts, one gathers the distinct impression that the strikingly different quality of profound deviance has elicited affects such as fear, threat, and shame, which, together with ignorance about its etiology, have substantially influenced treatment approaches. One favored "solution" was to isolate the extreme psychological deviant from his fellow man, often under conditions of total degradation and humiliation. Mental patients during the middle ages have been described as living like animals in a zoo and likened to inmates of leprosaria. Although animal-like exposure of patients to the elements ceased some time ago, until quite recently, living conditions in mental institutions were well characterized by the oft-cited "snake pit" metaphor.

To be sure, periods of "reform" and humanization of living conditions, associated with names such as Pinel in France and Dorothea Lynde Dix and Clifford Beers in this country, have occurred. However, some have argued (Foucoult, 1965; Greenblatt & Levinson, 1965) that certain reforms have served only to perpetuate patient isolation. Thus, predominant isolation from society and unfortunate living conditions have remained central to the destiny of the hospitalized mentally ill. Indeed, many believe that the major single objective of the Joint Commission on Mental Illness and Health, was to "slay the dragon" (see Chapter 2) of the large mental hospital and its presumed debilitating effects.

Recently, much interest has been directed to the nature of the mental hospital and the effects of its structure and organization on residents (Goffman, 1961; Scheff, 1966; Colarelli & Siegal, 1968; Rubenstein & Lasswell, 1966). Among the most penetrating and provocative of these analyses is the essay by Goffman (1961), who points to the dehumanizing, custodial, and defeatist orientation of many such settings. It is as if the total institution is, in the social-psychological sense, a burial ground where people are maintained but cease to exist in meaningful ways. Colarelli and Siegel (1966) graphically depict this view:

> His [the patient's] need to be protected, fed, and cared for gives institutional man his value. It is only natural that in such an institution the inmate's humanness increasingly diminishes. Who he is, what he is, his individual hopes, and problems and concerns recede into the background; he becomes an object—an object who fits into a routine, a bureaucratic pattern—to be cared for like any other object. As long as he remains in this role of the cared-for object and as long as the institution's staff members are willing to be caretakers, the cogs of the machine mesh and the intricate balance is maintained. The machine grinds on. Life, time, space and human experience become undifferentiated [p. iii].

Variations on the foregoing theme have been developed by other writers. For example, both Scheff (1966) and Braginsky *et al.* (1969) see the mental hospital patient as effectively playing the role that society and the institution set up for him as weak, compliant, peculiar, helpless, and committed to an essentially irreversible course of ineffectuality. Similarly, Rubenstein and Lasswell (1966) describe hospital inmates as individuals with chronic histories of lost power struggles in life, whose powerlessness and hopelessness is totally affirmed by the typical institutional setting, which leads to apathy and resignation,

Thus, the descriptive terms "custodially oriented" and "dehumanizing" often appear in current-day critiques of the large mental hospital, and the debilitating human consequences of such an atmosphere are cited with increasing frequency. A good deal of the current exploration of new treatment modalities for the profoundly ill rests on the foregoing view of the traditional mental hospitals, and is designed to overcome the perceived stagnating, dehumanizing consequences of such settings.

It is in no sense implied that improvement of mental hospital structures, however defined and however well carried out, constitutes an approach of choice in dealing with major mental illness. Elsewhere (Cowen & Zax, 1967; Cowen, 1967; Zax & Cowen, 1972) the point has been made, theoretically, that the best approach to profound psychological dysfunction is one that prevents its occurrence. As already noted, however, our limited present understanding of the etiology of schizophrenia and other forms of emotional dysfunction precludes our knowing whether prevention will come from advances in genetics, biochemistry and neurophysiology, environmental manipulation and control, or a combination of these approaches. Since we cannot, now, prevent profound disorder, and since, once established, such disorder resists enduring correction, the problem of how to help the mental hospital patient to a more gratifying and contributory life experience remains pressing.

C. New Approaches

One clearly discernible thrust in engaging this problem has been to try to break through, at many levels, the isolating and dehumanizing qualities of the traditional mental institution. To this end, the Joint Commission established a specific task-force to study and report on "new perspectives in mental patient care." The subgroup focused on three principal issues: (1) mechanisms to reduce and forestall institutionalization for mental illness, (2) increasing the effectiveness of mental hospitals, and (3) facilitating community readaptation following hospitalization for mental illness.

On the first point, the concept of the "community mental health center" has been proposed and implemented as one prospective way of averting hospitalization. Such centers seek to provide before-the-fact emergency services and to extend treatment facilities to more natural community settings, hopefully to reach and help people before the entrenchment of pathological conditions requires the more drastic alternative of institutionalization.

In pursuing the second issue, attempts to improve the effectiveness of mental hospitals have been made at several levels. Among the most basic of these are decisions about the very nature and location of mental institutions and more thoughtful consideration of how such elemental factors constrain or facilitate patient care. For example, to construct a 5000-bed mental hospital in a rural area, 50 miles from the nearest urban center, decidedly limits what can be done for patients. It doubtless hampers adequate staffing at all levels, restricts certain types of rehabilitative or therapeutic programming, isolates patients from the real world, inhibits access to and from a community surround, promotes a view of residents as alien, tainted, hopeless, and forgotten beings, and in general, fosters a management–custodial orientation to patient care.

The Joint Commission group, clearly perceiving these potential dangers, strongly recommended that "No further state hospitals of more than 1000 beds should be built, and not one patient should be added to any existing mental hospital already housing 1000 or more patients [p. 268]." They further recommended that future mental hospitals be located convenient to urban areas in order to maximize flexibility of programming and minimize both physical and psychological isolation, or stigmatization of the patient. An even more recent volume (Ullmann, 1967) indicates that when sizable samples of mental hospitals are studied, there are important relations among structural variables such as hospital size and patient-to-staff ratio, and indices of treatment effectiveness.

Recognition of the relationship between institutional structures and attitudes, on the one hand, and chronicity and dehumanization of the patient, on the other, underscores the importance of the question posed by Colarelli and Siegel (1966) as to how the "static helplessness" of the mental hospital patient can be changed. This question leads to a more detailed operational examination (Greenblatt & Levinson, 1965; Felix, 1967) of conditions of hospital living that foster static helplessness and fixate profound dysfunction. Locked wards, boredom, isolation from meaningful human contact, institutional garb, a foreordained, mandated, narrowly constricted living regimen, stereotypic negative labeling, a sense of powerlessness and lack of control over one's fate are all prospective contributing factors. Indeed, many attempts have been made in recent years to alleviate these long-standing, seemingly immutable bench marks of the mental hospital. Locked wards have been opened, flexibility of dress has been encouraged, and ventures in patient government have been undertaken. Efforts to replace custodial regimens with active treatment programs have been explored, and a variety of nonprofessionals, volunteers, and new types of helping-persons, have been introduced to hospital settings.

A good deal of the foregoing effort has developed within the framework of the "therapeutic community" (Jones, 1953; Jones, 1968; Rubenstein & Lasswell, 1966), an approach seen by some as particularly promising (Paul, 1969). In this same tradition, there has been an important, recent series of large-scale experiments to improve the conditions of the mental hospital and its patients (Fairweather, 1964; Colarelli & Siegal, 1966; Rubenstein & Lasswell, 1966; Ellsworth, 1968; Sanders, Smith, & Weinman, 1967). While there are differences among these projects in the populations served and in program specifics, collectively they have aimed at dramatic modification of mental hospital environments and ways of perceiving and interacting with patients that would avert the formerly drastic negative effects of the mental hospital on its residents. Factors emphasized in these programs include establishing genuinely therapeutic "total environments," reducing discontinuity between institution and community, according greater dignity and self-determination to the patient, and reconceptualizing personnel utilizations—both professional and nonprofessional. This is accomplished in ways that allow for increased, and far more functional human helping contact as opposed to largely custodial care. Paul (1969) regards this development as one of two currently extant ones that hold promise for the chronic mental patient. The second approach he cites has similar long-range objectives, but very different procedures and operations. This latter approach is based on behavior modification and the establishment of token economies involving contingency management of social behavior (Ayllon, 1963; Allyon & Azrin, 1969; Davison, 1969).

Increasingly, we have come to recognize that many mental hospitals are set up as if human beings existed as distinct, nonoverlapping types—the sick and the well—when in fact, mental illness, certainly in its earlier manifestations, tends to be *more or less* debilitating. Accordingly, many patients remain full-time in total institutions, usually not because their disability demands this, but because it is the only pigeon-hole available. In the main, we have failed to capitalize on patients' intact capacities and existing resources and have placed them in settings that encourage further regression rather than productivity within their potential.

With reference to the third issue addressed by the Joint Commission task force, recent developments in patient care have aimed at correcting deficiencies in community care. The day hospital, which accommodates the patient during working hours and allows him to spend evenings and weekends at home, is a case in point. During his time at the hospital, the patient receives treatment and acquires work and social skills. Conversely, the night hospital, based on a similar philosophy and underlying objectives, is geared to patients who, despite significant dysfunction, are capable of working and meeting everyday responsibilities of living; treatment and support are available to the patient during the evening hours. Both day and night hospitals pay heed to real individual differences among patients. Each offers the following advantages: reduced hospital–community discontinuity; minimized negative labeling or stigmatization; supported spheres of competence; open access-lines to home, community, and the outside world; and a move away from the potential debilitation caused by the total hospital environment.

A variety of evolving after-care programs also aim at early restoration of patients to the community and avoidance of the sick–well dichotomy that results from confining patients, who do not require such facilities, to mental hospitals. After-care programs include those that try to provide enough support to allow patients to function adequately outside the hospital as, for example, use of services provided by an outpatient clinic associated with the hospital, and transitional, sheltered environments. Among the latter, foster family placement is designed for patients who might otherwise languish in the hospital environment because they either have no home to return to or because they are not welcome at home. Foster placement allows the patient to readapt under conditions that offer some psychological support.

Another after-care modality that has attracted recent widespread interest is the "half-way house" (Fairweather, Sanders, Maynard, & Cressler, 1969; Rausch & Rausch, 1968). The Fairweather *et al.* program, a particularly interesting one, will be reviewed briefly later. The transitional "half-way" setting is for recovering patients who have progressed to the point where communal living with similar patients, backstopped by some professional consultation and services, holds additional therapeutic potential. As in the foster home, the half-way house removes the patient from the institution and offers some built-in protection and support. For some patients, it offers a needed privacy and independence not found in the foster home. Moreover, the fact that the constituency of the half-way house consists exclusively of ex-patients conveys a sense of kinship, companionship, and understanding that, for many, can be provided only by others who have lived through and shared a specific stressful life experience.

D. Conclusions

To summarize briefly what we have covered so far, we can state several important general conclusions. First, schizophrenia and other functional psychoses have been, and continue to be, the most perplexing behavior disorders known to man. Second, our cumulative record in advancing understanding and treatment has been poor. Third, the aura of mystery that shrouds these disorders and the manifestly extreme behavior they entail, elicit reactions such as shame, fear and threat in those who come into contact with them. Partly as a result of this, handling of such individuals has been isolating, dehumanizing, and custodial. Finally, as suggested, the struggle to cope effectively with extreme psychological dysfunction is proceeding on many fronts. For those with evolved and rooted disabilities, who have found their way into the mental hospital, much of this effort centers around programs designed to circumvent the debilitating consequences of the total institution. This effort has led to experimentation with programs and treatment modalities that share the objectives of reducing institution–community discontinuity, altering preconceived notions about patients, fostering active treatment approaches as opposed to resigned, custodial care, increasing patient self-determination; harnessing existing patient resources, and subverting the apathy and dehumanization of institutional settings.

While there can be little doubt about the depth and complexity of major mental illness or about the obvious need for prevention rather than repair, much of what can be done for those whose illness is already a here-and-now problem depends on human interest and resources—both of which have been woefully lacking for chronic hospitalized patients. The present study is addressed to this lacuna and seeks to provide a model for large-scale infusion of a new type of helping-person into the mental patient's world of helplessness and despair. The issue it poses is the extent to which energetic, enthusiastic, and devoted human involvement from the outside world can serve as a corrective for the chronic debilitation of mental hospital living. However, there is no illusion that such programming can *solve* the problems of major mental illness.

II. MANPOWER CONSIDERATIONS

A. The General Problem

In the past decade, mental health planners have become keenly aware of the tremendous shortages of manpower in the helping professions (Albee, 1959, 1963, 1966, 1967a, 1969; Arnhoff, Rubenstein, & Spiesman, 1969). Surveys such as those by Albee (1959) indicate that, in the professions of psychiatry, clinical psychology, social work, and psychiatric nursing, these shortages run from 25 to 75% below standards for minimal care. Moreover, extrapolations suggest that this disparity will become more severe in the future. More specific elements of this overall bleak forecast can be identified as follows: Our ability to train mental health professionals currently lags behind those interested in entering the field. We are also in a period of rapidly broadening redefinition of the scope of abnormal psychology with parallel increases in demand upon the professional for his scarce time (Zax & Cowen, 1972). Increasingly, the professional is called upon to help with social problems such as delinquency, urban unrest, cultural impoverishment, and curtailed education, each being a significant new challenge that in prior times would not have fallen within his domain. Activities directed toward the resolution of such problems will require considerable professional time. Because of limited professional resources, these new functions will compete with traditional activities for his scarce time.

B. The Need for New Approaches

The implications of the preceding analysis, discouraging though they may be, are even more complicated. For example, the limited existing resources of the mental health fields are unevenly distributed (Cowen & Zax, 1967; Zax & Cowen, 1972), following the ironic rule that "where help is most needed it is least available." Currently, the poor suffer the clearest application of this rule. However, it applies equally well to other segments of society, including those living in rural settings, and inmates of large mental hospitals. Such groups often fall, functionally, outside the scope of active, effective mental health intervention. As a result, many of their members must either fend for themselves or languish custodially in public institutions for prolonged periods of time. Thus, key professional positions remain chronically unfilled in many settings because we lack adequate professional manpower.

These facts highlight the need to formulate alternative conceptualizations about "cause and cure" of disorder and to explore innovative techniques for more effective delivery of helping services. The problems facing the mental health professions today far transcend those of the mental hospital inmate, and they are sufficiently pressing as to demand the formulation of such alternatives. As has been suggested elsewhere (Zax & Cowen, 1972), these alternatives must be developed both at the global and the specific levels. The methods and objectives of primary prevention illustrate the global approach; by contrast, using new manpower sources and redeploying existing resources may advance more delimited program objectives for certain target groups.

C. Recent Approaches to the Problem

Among the approaches that have gained recent attention as prospective solutions to existing mental health problems, is the use of a variety of nonprofessional workers in diverse mental health roles and settings. Not only is such use designed to cope with the practical exigencies created by gaping professional manpower shortages, but it is justifiably based on program effectiveness data (Sobey, 1970). The ingredients that are required for one human being to be helpful to another are not exclusive attributes of the professional. On the contrary, there are situations in which the nonprofessional, for a variety of reasons, may be *more* effective than the professional. Accordingly, the consideration and establishment of programs using nonprofessionals in mental health roles has increased many-fold in the past several years (Harris, 1966; Cowen, 1967; Arnhoff *et al.*, 1969; Grosser, Henry, & Kelly, 1969; Guerney, 1969; Sobey, 1970).

One cannot help being impressed by the rapid growth and unusual diversity of this development in terms of the individuals who have functioned as helpers, the groups with whom they have worked, the roles they have carried out, and the agencies and settings in which their activities have taken place. Even a brief overview of this development will illustrate its breadth and complexity.

D. Nonprofessionals as Mental Health Workers

Nonprofessional mental health workers have varied markedly with respect to such factors as age, socioeconomic status, prior background and experience, education, and social position. Many student groups have been used as helping-persons, including college undergraduates, high school and junior high school students, and even elementary-school children. Housewives, retired people, indigenous neighborhood workers, ex-convicts, ex-addicts or ex-mental-hospital inmates, hard-core delinquents and teenage youths, hospital attendants, parents, teachers, and welfare and enforcement workers have also been used. The groups with whom these helpers have worked have been equally varied: institutionalized mental hospital patients; clients of child guidance centers, community mental health centers, out-patient clinics and social service agencies; court cases; school children; inner-city residents; and women seen through pregnancy or well-baby clinics.

The decision to use nonprofessionals implies an emphasis on human and experiential factors as potential helping resources rather than the educational and intellective qualifications that we have traditionally emphasized. In practice, the amount of training given to nonprofessionals has ranged from virtually none to several years of essentially full-time preparation (Rioch, 1967). The nature and extent of training is determined by such factors as the conceptual orientation of the trainers, the job activities envisioned, and the life circumstances and major problems of the target groups. Among existing programs using nonprofessionals there are those that: (1) rely heavily upon a committed human relationship without being tied to specific techniques; (2) seek to train the nonprofessional to assume some delimited aspect of the professional's traditional functions (e.g., diagnosis or therapy); (3) utilize the life experience and style of the helper in working with concrete, everyday problems of those he serves; and (4) are based on specific methodologies, such as behavior modification, applied in particular ways with target-group members. The point has been made, for example (Sarason & Ganzer, 1969; O'Connor & Rappaport, 1970; Rappaport & O'Connor, 1970), that behavior modification approaches are eminently teachable and operational, and therefore comparatively easy, even for the untrained to master. Guerney's recent volume (1969) describes a number of specific behavior modification programs using nonprofessionals—parents, teachers, and peers—as change agents with diverse groups including school children, autistic children, acting-out adolescents, and mental hospital patients.

Its brevity notwithstanding, the preceding review attests to the tremendous range of efforts to find effective helping roles for nonprofessionals. This development is in understandable response to unmet social need and, as such, its active exploration, on many fronts, seems entirely justified. However, it would be an oversimplification, as several observers have noted (Reiff, 1967; Albee,

1969; Zax & Cowen, 1972), to assume that massive augmentation of the ranks of nonprofessionals will, itself, resolve major mental health problems of the time. *How* such workers are used is likely to be a more important question than *the number* used. Also, the harshest of all tests is the empirical one, which will be answered only by evaluation data deriving from programs in which nonprofessionals serve. Unfortunately, in the frenetic early surge to develop operational programs using nonprofessionals, rigorous research evaluation was largely bypassed.

III. NEW MANPOWER UTILIZATIONS IN THE MENTAL HOSPITAL

In all of its domains, the mental health field is currently being pushed to reexamine traditional manpower utilizations. There are few sectors of the field at large in which the dearth of manpower is felt as acutely as it is in the mental hospital. Arnhoff and Speisman (1969) point out that despite impressive absolute increases in professional mental health manpower in the helping fields since World War II, there are, ironically, *fewer* professionals on the staffs of state hospitals today than there were several decades ago. Whether this fact mirrors the nature of the institutions themselves (Ullmann, 1967), or the stark difficulties and unremitting disappointments that seem intrinsic to work with mental hospital inmates is of less concern than is the need perceived by those who would go beyond mere custodial maintenance, to explore viable alternatives. Reconceptualization and restructuring of total institutions, as illustrated in the previous section, is one such alternative. In this section, we shall discuss another alternative—the redeployment of people, including new uses of manpower, such as nonprofessionals, in ways that materially increase the human and humanizing contacts of the mental hospital patient.

A. Programs Using Nonprofessionals

1. THE HARVARD–RADCLIFFE PROGRAM

Among the early influential programs that systematically tapped the new breed of nonprofessional helping person for work with mental hospital patients was one established by Harvard and Radcliffe undergraduates with chronic patients in the Metropolitan State Hospital in Boston (Umbarger, Dalsimer, Morrison, & Breggin, 1962). During the 7-year period covered by their report (1954–1961), over 2000 student volunteers from Boston-area schools participated in many direct contacts and service functions with hospital inmates.

Companionship programs with adult and child patients, campaigns to improve the physical appearance and attractiveness of heretofore drab hospital wards, work as case-aides, participation in the establishment of half-way houses in which students and patients lived together, and a variety of special programs in teaching music, crafts, or foreign languages were among these. Whereas the initial account by Umbarger *et al.* (1962) was a clinical-descriptive summary of the program, with observations and impressions of its vitality, subsequent reports on the project have been more objectively oriented. For example, Greenblatt and Kantor (1962) indicate that program patients from a "withdrawn" ward demonstrated better conceptual organization and were behaviorally less withdrawn than those in the control wards.

In a more striking report, Beck, Kantor, and Gelineau (1963) point to the fact that 37% of a 120-patient sample seen by student volunteers was discharged from the hospital—a figure that compared favorably to the 3% discharge base-rate for the institution. Given the typical nature of institutional outcomes, this is an encouraging finding, even though the program patients were less chronic than the hospital controls to whom they were compared.

2. THE CONNECTICUT VALLEY PROGRAM

The student companion program, established in 1958 at the Connecticut Valley State Hospital (Holzberg, 1963; Holzberg & Gewirtz, 1964; Holzberg, Whiting, & Lowy, 1964; Holzberg & Knapp, 1965; Holzberg, Knapp, & Turner, 1967), has been another influential one. Utilizing the Harvard model, this program extended it by adding several research dimensions which evaluated program effects on both students and patients. Student volunteers were recruited from Abnormal Psychology classes, for patient-companionship activities. The role of professionals in the program was to provide support, supervision, and some training for the students. Evaluation of the program, which included hundreds of volunteers over the years, focused more on student reactions and attitude changes than on the patients. Positive changes in student attitudes and knowledge of mental illness, increases in self-acceptance, and reduction in severity of moral judgments took place as a result of program participation. Preliminary assessment of change in patients assigned to the program indicates some improvement in about 70%. The view has thus been expressed that the Connecticut Valley student companionship program simultaneously benefited patients, student volunteers, and the institution (Holzberg *et al.*, 1967).

The conviction that the early Connecticut Valley State Hospital Program was useful prompted formalization of a mechanism to permit college students to serve as helping persons in all state hospitals within the Connecticut system. As a result, the Connecticut State Department of Mental Hygiene established a Summer Service Corps, which attracts approximately 100 college students, for

8-week periods during the summer, to work as helpers with patients. A description of this program and a view of how it has worked are presented in a recent report by Scheibe, Kulik, Hersch, and La Macchia (1969). Although there was a sharp (25%) reduction in the number of hospitalized patients during the program period, there is no evidence that this is specifically due to the program. The authors believe, however, that students helped to improve communication among patients, increased interaction levels, and, in general, "softened up" hard-core chronic patients. A secondary program benefit is that a high percentage (60%) of student participants has gone on to mental health careers.

3. POSER'S STUDY

Although no attempt will be made here to review systematically or comprehensively all student volunteer programs, one recent, extremely important investigation (Poser, 1966) will be considered in greater detail because of its close parallel to the present study. This challenging investigation set out to compare the effectiveness of experienced mental health professionals with that of untrained female college undergraduates, as group leaders with chronic, hospitalized, adult, male schizophrenics. Few student leaders had even taken a single course in psychology and none had expressed interest in pursuing a future career in mental health. They were merely hired as part-time employees to do a specific job. By contrast, the psychiatrists and social workers were well trained with considerable prior mental health experience and specific experience with chronic schizophrenics.

The prime objective of the program was to foster verbal and social interaction among patients, using regularly scheduled group meetings as the vehicle for promoting such behavior. The professionals were given free reign in pursuing this objective. The students were simply oriented with respect to overall program aims and urged to do what they considered necessary and appropriate to further them.

The patient sample used in the investigation was clearly defined, relatively homogeneous, and sizable. It consisted largely of chronic schizophrenic patients with an average of 14 years confinement in a mental hospital, of which at least the last three had been consecutive. A total of 343 patients participated in the study, with assignment, following careful matching procedures, to one of three conditions: a no treatment (control) group, student-led groups and professional-led groups. There were 10 patients in each of the 13 student ($N = 130$) and 15 professional groups ($N = 150$), plus 63 controls. Contact was extensive between leaders and their groups, whether professional or nonprofessional. Meetings were held weekdays for 1 hour, over a 5-month period. Thus the experimental groups logged more than 100 sessions each.

a. Program Effects

Program effects were evaluated via a comprehensive test battery, individually administered to each patient before the study began and again after it ended. The battery included six objectively scored performance measures, widely used to evaluate hospitalized patients, reflecting psychomotor, perceptual, and verbal behavior. Among these were tests of word association, tapping speed, and reaction time. Although there were some preexperiment differences among groups on several of the measures, such differences were partialed out statistically, using covariance techniques, so that the groups could, in effect, be said to have begun from comparable starting points.

The findings are instructive. Undifferentiated comparison of combined-treatment groups (i.e., those seen by professionals or nonprofessionals) versus controls demonstrated significant differences on the criterion measures favoring the experimental groups. Thus, group contact, whatever its form, was beneficial. Patient improvement, however, was not equal across the two types of treatment groups. Surprisingly, those seen by student leaders showed *greater* improvement than those seen by professionals. This was directionally so for five of the six criterion measures and the differences favoring student-led groups were statistically significant on three of these (verbal fluency, reaction time, and tapping speed). A follow-up, 3 years later, with a small sample of patients who had participated in student-led groups demonstrated that the positive changes were largely stable over time.

b. Imperfections

However, there are several important flaws in Poser's study. For example, the findings are somewhat confounded by a higher patient drop-out rate in the student-led groups than in professionally led groups. One can also question the use of *test* criteria of patient change as opposed to relevant behavioral change, such as discharge from the hospital. Still another point of contention is that most professional group leaders were males, whereas student leaders were young, attractive females working with male patients. Critics of the study have seized upon these points. For example, Rosenbaum (1966) argues that the improvement of patients was due only to the warmth and humaneness of these young, vibrant people, and this should not be mistaken for psychotherapy. In the view of the present authors, how we label the source of change seems far less important than the *fact* of constructive change in profoundly and chronically disturbed individuals, ostensibly unreachable by other available methods for an average of 14 preceding years. A comment on this point bears citation here: "Given the known difficulties of effectuating positive change in human behavior by any means, to insist that change is true change only when it follows psychotherapy or interventions by trained professionals, is a luxury we can ill afford [Cowen, 1967, p. 427]!"

c. *Overall Effectiveness*

While Poser's findings can justifiably be challenged on several counts, there is little basis for explaining why patients seen by students should have shown significantly *greater* improvement than those seen by professionals, unless one looks beyond the oft-cited intellective, training, and experiential attributes of mental health professionals in trying to identify critical change factors. Poser's results put before us the possibility that *human* and *stylistic* factors may be vastly underrated as variables capable of promoting positive change in the mental hospital patient. The generalization value of Poser's study, as he himself recognizes it, is limited by factors such as setting, patient sample, group leaders, and criterion measures employed. Its value comes less from the generalizations that he establishes and more from the manner in which his findings force critical reexamination of prior and seemingly immutable "dos and don'ts" of mental hospital patient care. In that sense, it should encourage energetic, further exploration of flexible new uses of nonprofessionals in the mental hospital, in particular, and in the mental health fields more generally. The questions of how one human being provides interpersonal help for another and whether this help is something that can best be provided by mental health professionals remain very much open. Such questions are central to the focus of the present project.

B. Overview and Future Prospects

Pressing social need and the promising results of early programs have converged to spark a rapid proliferation of student volunteer programs in mental hospitals. From modest beginnings in the mid-fifties, there has been a near exponential increase in such programs in the ensuing years. Whereas in 1956, there were fewer than 30 colleges and universities sponsoring student volunteer programs, it has been estimated (NIMH, 1968) that during the academic years 1955–1966, 8000 students from more than 300 schools served as volunteers in programs for mental hospital patients. These figures are probably underestimates of the actual number. Today, many colleges and universities, either formally or informally, sponsor programs in which students carry out mental health-relevant functions in diverse settings, including particularly those for patients experiencing profound psychological upset. The general increase in college enrollments, the corresponding rise in the number of undergraduates majoring in psychology, and the growing cry for relevance currently heard on the college campus, together suggest that the use of college students in helping programs will continue to accelerate in coming years.

C. Nonprofessionals Other Than College Students

The base of this discussion can be broadened to include use of nonprofessionals other than college students as helping persons with mental hospital patients. Findings with other groups of nonprofessionals support those deriving from student volunteer programs. A number of these investigations (Appleby, 1963; Mendel & Rapport, 1963; Carkhuff & Truax, 1965) provided specific training for nonprofessionals, typically hospital aides or attendants, to allow them to assume segments of heretofore exclusively professional roles, as, for example, individual and group therapy with chronic patients. The aim of these programs was to develop more active treatment interventions for those who would otherwise languish unattended. Their findings suggest that nonprofessionals function effectively as change agents and do about as well as professionals in this regard. In the study by Carkhuff and Truax (1965), for example, eight 10-patient groups were seen twice weekly for several months by five nonprofessional lay therapists who had been given focused, time-limited training. Patients seen by nonprofessionals were judged to have improved significantly more than comparable untreated controls on a variety of ward-behavior measures. An even more challenging finding was reported by Anker and Walsh (1961) who compared chronic mental patients who had participated in nonprofessionally led "activity groups" with a similar patient group seen in group therapy by professionals. Patients seen by nonprofessionals improved more in rated total adjustment, motility, communication, and cooperation than did those seen in group therapy by the professionals.

1. THE WARD H PROJECT

Comprehensive projects that transcend teaching delimited professional techniques to nonprofessionals have also been reported. These projects have been stimulated by the sense of futility generated by custodially oriented hospitals. The Ward H project of the Topeka State Hospital (Colarelli & Siegel, 1966) exemplifies this approach. The active agent in this program was the mental hospital aide who has characteristically functioned as the lowest-ranking member of the hospital staff—i.e., as an arm of the "responsible" professional, carrying out the least significant and least demanding patient-care activities. The key to the Ward H approach is found in the following statement: "Instead of making the aides middlemen, let's make them headmen. Let's give them the patients and tell them they're totally responsible for those patients and their treatment. If the aides want help from the staff, they can ask for it, but the treatment is up to them and we confidently expect results [Colarelli & Siegel, 1966, p. v]." Aides were thus given responsibility for systematic observation of patients—formulating and implementing treatment plans, record keeping, scheduling of activities and establishing extra-hospital contacts, as, for example, with the patient's family or the community at large. To achieve these ends, a number of heretofore sacrosanct hospital regulations were scrapped and aides were permitted to do such things as return to the ward after working hours, eat with patients on the ward, initiate money-making projects with patients, take patients for car rides to various amusements, or invite them to their homes. Aides were given formal and informal training in the psychopathology of schizophrenia and in the "ego-boundaries" approach to treatment. The Ward H program did not develop smoothly from the start. Indeed, at the outset, there were morale problems, periods of heightened anxiety, and resignations of project personnel. These problems, however, dimished over time and the program functioned well in its later phases.

The Ward H project, involving 36 chronic schizophrenic patients, took 4 years and was researched at multiple levels. For example, the frequent occurrence of certain types of critical ward incidents in the 3 months immediately preceding and following the program were compared. Off-grounds passes increased by about 300% from preprogram levels; eight times as many patients had job assignments; and the rate of assault incidents dropped to 10% of its original level. While discharge rates on Ward H were approximately the same as for the rest of the hospital, readmission rates were about one-seventh of the overall hospital figure. Supportive results, showing improvement of the Ward H subjects over controls, were also found in results of a standardized psychodiagnostic test battery including the Wechsler–Bellevue intelligence scale, an object sorting test, figure drawing, and the Rorschach inkblot test. Particularly significant among observed patient changes, was the greater ability of the Ward H patient to behave in socially acceptable ways and an increase in his internal resources, making him more independent.

Based on both observational and test data, important behavioral changes were also found among aides—especially greater spontaneity, involvement, confidence, maturity, and autonomy. The success of the Ward H project is due to the fact that ". . . a social system was permitted to evolve which supported and nurtured a growth inducing relationship between psychiatric aides and tragically dehumanized patients [Colarelli & Siegel, 1966, p. 205]."

2. THE FORT MEADE PROJECT

A project, similar to Ward H in objectives and implementation, was the Fort Meade investigation reported by Ellsworth (1968). Both programs sought to harness the therapeutic potential of the aide and both emphasized increasing the spontaneity of aide–patient interaction and the genuine involvement of the aide in making critical decisions. Unlike the Topeka group, the Fort Meade aides did not receive formal training. It was thought that such training would, deleteriously, give the aides the impression that they lacked requisite helping skills. Thus, training at Fort Meade was informal and centered around the clinical interaction. It was based upon clear communication of role expectancies by available role-models, immediate feedback on aide performance, and palpable rewards, such as increased status and assignment to aides of decision-making responsibilities. Simply stated, the Fort Meade group tried to enhance the aide's usefulness by enlarging his role rather than by retraining him using traditional classroom, seminar or workshop approaches.

A total of 336 male schizophrenic patients, 122 experimentals (Es) and 214 controls (Cs), participated in the Fort Meade experiment. Both Es and Cs were divided into three subgroups, reflecting different levels of chronic dysfunction. The E and C conditions were comparable with respect to: patient characteristics, the degree to which medication and activity groups were used, decision-making processes for patient discharge, and policies on new admissions. The E group had smaller ward units and a higher aide–staff ratio. It also had progressively differentiated wards—"closed," "open," and "discharge"—through which patients advanced as a function of actual behavioral change. The key differences between the E and C conditions were increased aide–patient interaction and greater aide autonomy and responsibility in the treatment process for Es. For example, at the start of the study, E-aides spent an average of 14% of their time in off-ward interactions with patients. By the end, that figure had jumped to 69%.

The experiment covered a 30-month period and a patient follow-up, both within and outside the hospital, was conducted for 6 years afterward. The prime within-hospital criteria used in the evaluation were ward behavior measures, length of stay, and discharge rates. Interestingly, discharge rates rose significantly for *both* the E and C groups, suggesting that the study had hospital-wide impact. On most within-hospital measures, Es did better than Cs, particularly among *more* chronic patients. Overall, including both Es and Cs, about two-thirds of the sample was discharged at some time during the study, and about one-half achieved "significant release" (i.e., followed by 12 or more consecutive months in the community). In the E group, however, release rates were higher and return rates lower. Seven critical outcome variables significantly differentiated the two groups. In comparison to the C groups, Es had better behavioral adjustment, fewer days hospitalized, higher discharge rates, a greater "significant release" ratio, better social adjustment outcomes, superior work adjustment outcomes, and a more favorable discharge status at the 6-year follow-up point. All differences except the last were highly significant; the last was significant only when comparing *chronic* Es with *chronic* Cs. Differences between the E and C groups were greater as one moved from the relatively more acute to the relatively more chronic levels. Based on these striking findings, Ellsworth (1968) concluded:

> . . . the results of the experimental program can be explained most easily by stating that when a treatment program uses the resources of a large number of its personnel in a *meaningful* way, the program will be successful. If on the other hand, the significant roles are restricted to the professional staff, results will be less distinctly successful [p. 165].

3. THE PHILADELPHIA STATE HOSPITAL PROJECT

A rather different approach to chronic patient treatment, based on another type of innovative nonprofessional manpower use, is reported in the Philadelphia State Hospital Project (Sanders, 1967; Sanders, Smith, & Weinman, 1967). This program used a socioenvironmental therapy approach that sought to promote social interaction among chronic patients by creating a milieu that increased both demands and opportunities for social functioning. A key problem in establishing such a program, as Sanders (1967) observes, is its heavy personnel requisites. To fill these needs, the Philadelphia group decided to recruit and train college graduates with no prior experience in mental health. Their training objectives included instilling humanitarian, treatment-oriented attitudes, learning about the hospital culture, and becoming familiar both with the tenets and procedures of the socioenvironmental method. This training, including didactic, discussion, and practicum components, required nearly a year.

The basic hospital restructuring included humanizing the living conditions of patients, promulgating the concept of a therapeutic community in patients and staff, creating a variety of experiences in social living, and developing a framework for patient government and self-determination. Patient training in a variety of social behaviors, individual, and group corrective experiences was entrusted largely to the nonprofessionals—the "social interaction therapists." The program rested on the assumption that massive increases in opportunities and demands for social interaction, led by the new nonprofessionals, would lead to more favorable outcomes in chronic schizophrenic patients.

Nearly 300 chronic male and female patients participating in the investigation were assigned to one of four conditions. The three experimental conditions varied in the degree to which interaction was built into the program (i.e., "minimally," "partially," and "maximally"). The fourth was a control group. The results of the study are reasonably complicated. For example, whereas the maximally structured group showed greatest improvement in spontaneous social behavior, there were no significant differences among conditions in posttreatment status. In general, the older, more chronic patients, particularly those in the maximally structured condition, profited most from the program, both in improved social adjustment and in psychiatric status. Apparently, younger, less chronic patients were upset by the demands for interpersonal closeness inherent in the approach. A 3-year follow-up indicated that discharged program patients, especially those in the more structured conditions, had adjusted more adequately to the community than did their control peers. Again, older, more chronic patients surpassed younger ones in all areas of community adjustment. Thus, the lowest return rates to the hospital were found among older, chronic patients who had participated in the maximally structured condition. While the findings of this study are complex, with subtle nuances and complicated interactions, the authors nevertheless conclude (Sanders *et al.*, 1967): "Clearly, socioenvironmental treatment offers hope of release and community adjustment to a large group of chronic mental patients previously destined to spend their remaining years in mental hospital wards [p. 301]." This program thus combines a new treatment conceptualization with an innovative use of nonprofessional manpower.

4. THE FAIRWEATHER PROJECT

A related project is cited here, even though it is based more on changing the patient's role and status than on new uses of nonprofessional manpower. The need to overcome the sense of powerlessness and helplessness that so often characterizes chronic patients has frequently been cited (Rubenstein & Lasswell, 1966). This point is central to the work of Fairweather and his associates (Fairweather, 1964, 1967; Fairweather *et al.*, 1969), which at its core, seeks to create, for patients, role behaviors that are consonant with the demands and realities of community living. In the earlier phases of his project (Fairweather, 1964), this objective was broached by creating autonomous, responsible, patient-led task groups. When the effects of this intervention as a treatment method were compared with a traditional hospital care approach, the results indicated that the autonomous group showed greater social activity and heightened participation in group events, even for chronic patients. Morale improved, acceptance of responsibility was greater, as were patient concerns about their fellows. In other words, patients became capable of caring for each other, making realistic and important life decisions, and an adequate, semiautonomous, hospital adjustment. Staff morale also improved noticeably. Upon release from the hospital, patients from the autonomous groups had more favorable immediate work records and social adjustments. The major drawback, however, was that the gains did not hold up for long when the supportive, within-hospital structure was no longer available. Thus nearly 60% of those discharged from both the autonomous and traditional groups, returned to the hospital within 6 months.

The disappointing recidivism data from this early study led Fairweather *et al.* (1969) to create a new type of extra-hospital setting: a small self-contained society within the larger community, where chronic patients could find a continuing supportive group situation that was no longer available to them in the earlier studies after discharge. From among patients who volunteered for the new lodge-type community, both an experimental (E) group, which actually became part of it, and a matched control (C) group, which remained in the hospital, were selected. Cs participated in standard hospital after-care programs, involving family contacts and out-patient visits.

While many problems were encountered in setting-up this novel community, and a good deal of supervision was initially required, patient leadership emerged within several months. Patients assumed full responsibility for operating and governing the setting, including, for example, setting salary levels, determining allocations of money and resources, establishing discipline regulations, and setting up business operations. Not only did this new society prove workable, but in comparison with patients in more traditional hospital and after-care programs, members were shown to have enhanced self-esteem, superior employment records and, most important, lived longer periods in the community. The patient is a prospectively important treatment resource in dealing with the complex problems of major mental illness. This is suggested by Fairweather *et al.* (1969) ". . . the paramount implications of this study . . . is the urgent need to create new and more participative social statuses and roles for those members who only marginally belong to [society] . . . [p. 8]." This conclusion is consonant with the position taken, increasingly, by other workers in the area (Scheff, 1966; Rubenstein & Lasswell, 1966; Braginsky *et al.*, 1969).

IV. THE EFFECTIVENESS OF NONPROFESSIONALS

Several points in the preceding discussion deserve more explicit emphasis. The search for effective new treatment modalities for the chronically ill has led, in recent years, to dramatic increases in programs using new groups of nonprofessional helping agents, and those redeploying nonprofessionals previously involved in menial or custodial functions. Much of this thrust rests on a recognition that patients, once consigned to a mental hospital, are typically destined to remain there for prolonged periods. Thus, the development is but one manifestation of a broader effort to reach the functionally unreached and to humanize the interactions and life experiences of the mental hospital patient. Review of a number of programs of this emergent type, all using nonprofessionals, suggests that they have been useful, judged by the criterion of positive patient change. Since, in many instances, the patients in question were among the most chronic and least curable, the findings are all the more impressive.

A. Why Nonprofessionals Are Effective

1. QUALITIES OF THE NONPROFESSIONAL

The effectiveness of programs using nonprofessionals in the mental hospital has brought about speculation as to *what* makes them work (see Section V). One widely cited set of such factors (Poser, 1966; Rioch, 1966; Holzberg, 1966; Cowen, 1967; Cowen, Chinsky, & Rappaport, 1970) includes the qualities of enthusiasm, involvement, high motivation, and dedication that characterize the approach of many nonprofessionals in the clinical setting. The nonprofessional is challenged by the task, recognizing that the activities he will undertake have heretofore belonged exclusively to the highly trained professional. The college student particularly exemplifies this situation. As a late adolescent or young adult, often with a somewhat sheltered life history, the challenge of becoming an active agent in a real situation in the "real world" is valid and welcome in his search to establish identity as a mature, productive adult. As has been pointed out elsewhere (Cowen *et al.*, 1970), the cry for relevance so often echoed these days on college campuses and the wish to find alternatives to encapsulated "book-learning" situations are, for many students, well met through bona fide human service activity, of which mental hospital volunteer work is a good example. Whatever their source, attributes such as the vibrance and enthusiasm of nonprofessionals may be especially useful to patients who have been exposed, for long periods, to institutional settings characterized by a defeatist orientation and the care-objective of quietly maintaining the status quo. For such patients, the different and refreshing approach of the nonprofessional provides a new type of model and a meaningful potential link to a long-forgotten way of life. The nonprofessional may thus be seen as a catalyst in an otherwise imperceptibly slow process.

2. NONPROFESSIONAL APPROACH

Another element of a generalized "enthusiasm" hypothesis is that nonprofessionals may approach interpersonal helping situations, particularly those where professionals have been unsuccessful, such as in the state hospital, with a different, more positive, set of expectancies than those held by professionals. They are inclined, in their naive, refreshing simplicity, to see patients first as people rather than as the hopelessly and incurably ill. Professionals are sometimes shocked and upset by such an "oversimplified approach," which may even run counter to what the professional has been taught to do and expect. Perhaps, however, this refreshing approach is what some hospital patients require. Because the nonprofessional *expects* them to do so, patients may respond when spoken to or join groups and play games when invited. In this context, the writers are reminded of an illuminating incident that took place during the present study. One group, consisting largely of chronic, regressed patients, included a patient who had been totally mute for 10 years. The student leader, not realizing the implications of that fact, continued to talk to the patient and to invite him to respond. After a while, the patient began to go through the motions of participating in games and group activities remaining, however, mute. In the middle of one such session, while playing monopoly, the patient suddenly exclaimed—his first utterance in 10 years—"You landed on Atlantic Avenue and you owe me $22!"

Clearly, no matter how high the expectancy of the nonprofessional, and no matter how effective his behavior and entreaties, he will not be able to draw *all* patients into meaningful social interaction. Rather, the point of our argument is that people's behavior may, in some measure, relate to the expectancies that others hold for them. To the extent that the nonprofessional has more positive, optimistic expectancies than the professional, including the expectations of more normal prosocial behavior, a meaningful force toward encouraging such behavior exists.

3. LACK OF ORTHODOX TRAINING

Another attribute of the nonprofessional, which may promote positive patient change, is that he is less constrained than the professional by established rules of interaction and unimpeachable wisdoms about how troubled people are helped. Professional training teaches "correct versus incorrect," and "appropriate versus inappropriate" ways of interacting with patients. It is not clear that these so-called correct and appropriate ways are also effective ones. In the absence of lengthy formal training and the acquisition of a framework of regularities for patient interaction, the nonprofessional must grope for ideas that work and must depend more heavily upon natural wisdom, life experiences, and pragmatism. Thus, he is forced into far greater flexibility and more trial-and-error than is the professional.

In a field where we know so little about what *is* helpful for patients, perhaps this forced flexibility can uncover productive new approaches and can expand our currently limited repertoire of effective helping techniques. Whereas the professional may perceive the nonprofessional's behavior as unsophisticated, wrong, lacking precedent, and implausible, if he can endure such amateurish exploration in a relatively relaxed, unthreatened manner, there is much potentially to be learned about effective treatment of the profoundly ill. Zealous overguarding of professional prerogatives and patient-handling techniques may, in the final analysis, deter constructive change and growth in patients. This is not a one-sided argument, however. The exploratory approach of nonprofessionals will result in errors and create problems. On the other hand, the "house" of mental health, in particular those aspects of it that shelter the mental hospital patient, is presently far more plagued by errors of omission than those of commission.

4. SOCIAL DISTANCE HYPOTHESIS

A final concept advanced in an effort to understand the effectiveness of nonprofessionals as help agents is the so-called "social distance hypothesis" (Rioch, 1966; Chinsky & Rappaport, 1971; Cowen, 1967). This view is based on the assumption of a social status hierarchy, topped by mental health professionals. The position occupied by the professional has potential advantages and disadvantages. The advantages lie in the wisdom and authority often imputed to the expert, and in the fact that many individuals who require help feel considerable need to be seen by a person with high status and regard. Conversely, there are other individuals experiencing intrapersonal distress for whom the status, authority, and style of the expert are inhibiting or distasteful—sufficiently, in some cases, to thwart establishing an effective relationship and to impair meaningful communication. This danger has prompted development of an alternate approach in inner-city mental health programs built around the use of indigenous nonprofessionals (Reiff & Riessman, 1965). The indigenous worker shares the life experience of his ghetto clientele and speaks their language; his interaction style is consistent with that of the inner-city residents with whom he works. These group attributes win trust, provide entrées, and facilitate more effective rendering of services to the previously unreached.

Similarly many inmates of mental hospitals see themselves as belonging to a social plane other than that of the mental health professional. Thus, even if sufficient professional services were available, for many patients there would remain a style and communication chasm between themselves and professionals blocking effective treatment. In such cases, the nonprofessional, in a lower position in the social status hierarchy, may be more readily accepted and thus in a better position than professionals to establish meaningful contact with some patients. In short, he may serve as a more effective model than the professional.

B. Redeployment of Existing Nonprofessionals

Our discussion, thus far oriented to the new nonprofessional being introduced in mental hospital settings as a prospective change agent, can be profitably extended to redeployments of existing nonprofessional groups such as aides and attendants. As noted in Section III, D, such personnel have historically fallen into the pattern set by the system, i.e., to maintain patients and preserve the status quo. Brown, in her introduction to Ellsworth's volume, describes this orientation.

> Their [the aides'] duties include doing ward work or supervising patients doing it, and maintaining a quiet ward with the minimum of disturbance possible. Otherwise the attendants were likely to spend their time talking to each other, reading comic books, or trying to sustain their boredom until the end of shift or duty. Few of them attempted to interest patients in games or in any activity other than ward work. As a result, patients on many wards spent much of the day sitting listlessly looking into space, thus regressing farther both mentally and physically . . . . The care of patients was viewed primarily as that of custody, not treatment [Ellsworth, 1968, p. xiii].

As noted previously, recent programs such as those of Colarelli and Siegel (1966) and Ellsworth (1968) have broken away from this traditional passive-custodial model by giving aides bona fide treatment responsibilities, decision-making authority, and a stake in an active treatment program. Since aides are the people in a hospital with whom patients have most frequent daily contact, their attitudes and behaviors are critical in establishing an institutional atmosphere and in influencing patient change.

A recent conference on psychiatric rehabilitation (Kandel & Williams, 1964) sets the issue of utilization of nonprofessionals in mental hospitals in a worthwhile perspective. Several conference foci are reflected in the following statements from their work:

> . . . the present logistics of mental health services results in people's getting lost or pushed into a social Deepfreeze when in a mental hospital . . . institutional confinement is frequently anti-therapeutic and the present state hospital system, in particular, causes fear, discomfort, [and] degradation of the individual [pp. 12-13].

The "social Deepfreeze" is largely a consequence of overcrowded, dehumanizing conditions and manpower shortages that motivated using nonprofessionals. Even if sufficient professional manpower were available, how many useful skills would the professional have available? Perhaps, as we have already suggested, no more than the nonprofessionals, and in some instances fewer. The chronic patient suffering the effects of institutionalism needs something to draw him back into the social environment–into some meaningful social role. One possible approach to this end is to offer him a genuine human relationship in which he is upgraded rather than degraded. To maintain the phrase used by conference, if existing institutional structures for the care of the mentally ill constitute a "social Deepfreeze" is it not reasonable to hope that the patient may be helped by turning on a modicum of "social heat?"

C. Limits of the Nonprofessional

1. PREVENTION VERSUS CURE

While it is possible to generate enthusiasm for more widespread use of nonprofessional helping agents with mental hospital patients, it would be a serious error to think of this development as a panacea. Several of its limits should be kept firmly in mind. Among the most important of these is a conceptual one. Such programs, however effective, begin with already seriously disturbed patients. The case has been made that before-the-fact prevention is far more important than after-the-fact repair (see p. 5). Put in other terms, effective use of new nonprofessional manpower, however much it extends mental health helping resources to the functionally unreached, is less urgently needed than a reconceptualization of our approach to highly disordered behavior (Scheff, 1966). Our most effective future manpower utilizations will be the consequence rather than the determinant of innovative and adaptive conceptualizations.

2. NOVELTY OF THE SITUATION

The qualities of involvement, dedication, and positive expectancy that seemingly characterize the nonprofessional and are significant factors in promoting patient improvement, may be typical initial reactions of people who are excited and ego-involved in challenging new life situations. If this is true, then positive change in target individuals as a result of programs using nonprofessionals may primarily reflect program novelty and thus run the risk of dissipating as the novelty and challenge of the new situation decreases.

3. LACK OF DETAILED PROGRAM EVALUATION

Another reality factor that dampens excessive enthusiasm about evolving manpower utilizations, is that this development owes its existence to compelling social need and impressionistic evaluation by ego-involved observers. Though this has been largely inevitable, it is potentially misleading and dangerous. While there are exceptions, on the whole, it is fair to say that rigorous research evaluations of programs using nonprofessionals has been lacking. Rather, what we have is a "sense" of their workability and a logical rationale for further exploration. We do not clearly understand how such programs work when they do, nor have we carefully explored a number of pertinent questions beyond the immediately obvious one of: "Does a program using nonprofessionals work?" An example of such a question is: "Can we predict those patients who will take to, stay with, and profit from, human service programs staffed by nonprofessionals?" Many questions can, and must be raised about nonprofessionals and how their attitudes, personality make-up, and actions influence program outcomes. In the section to follow, a series of such questions central to this investigation, and their rationale, will be presented.

However, for the moment let it be emphasized that our intent in this project was to approach a network of basic questions about the use of nonprofessionals as helpers with mental hospital patients in a systematic, research-based way. The field has not lacked for pilot or demonstration programs using nonprofessionals, but it sorely needs a body of objectively grounded knowledge about such uses if we are to separate wheat from chaff and have a basis for developing new and more socially utilitarian programs.

V. HELPER ATTRIBUTES

The preceding sections have focused on the questions of whether nonprofessionals can function meaningfully in human service capacities, particularly with chronic mental hospital patients, and if so, what factors contribute to their effectiveness. While the tentative answer to the first question is affirmative, the contributing evidence comes from clinical observation and impressionism born of need, rather than from sound, systematic research findings. Even if "hard" affirming data were available, the question as to whether nonprofessionals are effective or not is an oversimplification. In the last analysis, the answer will not simply be "yes" or "no," but will reflect relationships among characteristics of the helper group, attributes of the individual helper, specific roles and functions being performed, target groups served, and settings in which services are rendered. A second basic purpose of the present investigation is to examine some of the latter issues through intensive study of the helping person—in this case the college-student volunteer. The growing use of college students as human-service personnel in mental hospitals, and their effectiveness in this role, underscores the importance of these issues. In the following section, four focal issues pertaining to the use of college-student volunteers are identified and developed. Each reflects an important area for further investigation in the present research.

A. Personality Attributes of the Effective Nonprofessional

At this time, we do not clearly understand the attributes of effective mental health *professionals.* Indeed, both Colby (1964) and Kiesler (1966) have observed that psychotherapy researchers have been led astray by the naive assumption that all therapists are alike. If this is true for professionals who share common elements of training, experience, viewpoint, and ethos, it is reasonable to assume that it applies many-fold to nonprofessionals, who are considerably more heterogenous. There is little reason to suppose that all nonprofessionals are equally effective in general, much less in terms of their work with different target groups and in different situations. The problem we faced in approaching this complex issue was to pick and choose from a variety of approaches, variables that logically or empirically gave promise of differentiating among more or less effective college student volunteers in the mental hospital. Our thinking in this matter was influenced by three prior lines of investigation bearing on the effectiveness of helping persons: those of Truax and Carkhuff (1967), Whitehorn and Betz (1954), and Goodman (1965, 1969).

1. TRUAX AND CARKHUFF

Truax and Carkhuff (1967) have identified three personality variables related to therapeutic effectiveness. These attributes are:

(1) *Accurate empathy:* defined as "the therapist's *sensitivity to current feelings* and his *verbal facility to communicate this understanding* in a language attuned to the client's current feelings [p. 46]";
(2) *Nonpossessive warmth:* by which "the therapist warmly accepts the patient's experience as part of that person, without imposing conditions . . . . It means accepting [the client] . . . as a person with human potentialities [p. 58]";
(3) *Genuineness or self-congruence:* where "the therapist is freely and deeply himself [p. 58]." Theoretically, these traits are *natural* ingredients in an individual's make-up (Rogers, 1957) and are presumed to exist differentially among college students.

Truax (1961) developed operational measures of these three characteristics based on rating scales used to evaluate short, 2- to 4-minute segments of therapeutic interactions. These measures have been applied to group sessions conducted by lay personnel with patient samples similar to the one used in this study (Carkhuff & Truax, 1965; Carkhuff, 1969a,b). Truax's findings (1961) suggested that the previously mentioned variables were significant interpersonal dimensions which related positively to successful outcomes with patients.

2. WHITEHORN AND BETZ

Another line of relevant research is in the work of Whitehorn and Betz (1954) who reported that certain psychiatric residents, designated "A's," were more successful in treating hospitalized schizophrenics than other residents, designated "B's." A-therapists were described by Betz (1962) as more frequently ascertaining "the personal meaning and motivation of the patient's behavior" and they "more frequently selected personality-oriented rather than psychopathology-oriented goals in the treatment of a particular patient [p. 44]." They were also more freely expressive and developed more trust in their patients than did B's.

Whitehorn and Betz (1954) found that A's differed significantly from B's on four occupational keys of the Strong Vocational Interest Blank (SVIB). A's were higher on the lawyer and certified public accountant keys while B's were higher on the printer, and mathematics and physical science teacher keys. Further analysis (Betz, 1962) indicated significant differences between the two groups on 23 of the 400 items of the SVIB. This finding, using 15 A and 11 B therapists, was duplicated at another clinic with a new sample of 46 physicians (Betz, 1962). Using these 23 items, Betz (1962) developed an "A–B Scale" which differentiated psychiatric residents successful in treating hospitalized schizophrenics from those less successful.

A later study by Lorr and McNair (1962), found that B therapists were more successful than A's in treating outpatient neurotics and character disorders. Several explanations for the differential effectiveness of A and B therapists with schizophrenics and neurotics have been proposed. Betz (1966), for example, suggested that A's use different problem-solving approaches. Shows and Carson (1965) found that B's were more field-independent, and thus less attuned to the patient than A's. Social class differences and degree of masculine interest have also been considered as possible sources of the observed differences between the two groups (Lorr & McNair, 1966). Other researchers (e.g., Carson, Harden, & Shows, 1964; Kemp, 1966; Berzins & Seidman, 1968, 1969) have suggested possible interactions between therapist-type (A versus B) and the different syndromes of neurotic and psychotic patients, to account for their differential effectiveness with different groups.

One possible reason for the success of A therapists with schizophrenics has been suggested by Tourney, Bloom, Lowinger, Schorer, Auld, and Grisell (1966). In a study of therapeutic interactions of psychiatric residents with schizophrenics and neurotics, they found that neurotics responded to therapist (T) technique, whereas, schizophrenics responded more to T affect. Independent ratings of positive feelings expressed by T were related to significant decreases in thought disorder, anxiety, hostility to others, and negative arousal in schizophrenic patients, and to significant increases in positive feelings expressed by the patients toward T and others. Neurotic patients showed similar trends, but, with the exception of positive feelings expressed toward T, these relations were less marked.

The conclusions of Tourney *et al.* (1966) are particularly interesting in view of the seemingly differential success of A versus B therapists. Neurotics may be helped more by the technique-oriented, less personal, more field-independent B-type therapists. Schizophrenics, being more influenced by the openness, warmth, and positive feelings of T rather than his technique, react more favorably to A-type therapists. The seemingly greater effectiveness of A-therapists with schizophrenics warrants further study and extrapolation to college student volunteers.

3. GOODMAN

A third approach to the study of the effective college-student volunteer is found in the work of Goodman (1965, 1969). Goodman has developed a structured behavioral technique to assess understanding, openness, and accepting-warmth. His procedure, known as the "Group Assessment of Interpersonal Traits (GAIT)" was used to screen undergraduate male applicants for a companionship program[1] (Goodman, 1965, 1969). In a simulated group situation, eight students are asked, individually and in turn, to disclose a personal problem. These problems are dealt with by any other group member. Using a "round-robin" sequence, each group member reveals a problem, comments on and tries to understand the problem posed by another student. At the end of a session, which typically takes about 1½ hours, ratings of each participant on the following dimensions are made by all students in the group and by more experienced observers: accepting-warmth, depression, quietness, openness, understanding, rigidity, and degree of tension expressed. An overall rating of "Best Counselor" is also obtained. Goodman combined the open, understanding, and accepting-warmth dimensions as a single measure of "Therapeutic Talent," a behaviorally derived measure that might relate to the effectiveness of the student as a group leader.

B. Comparisons of Volunteers and Nonvolunteers

In the present study, we are also concerned with the extent to which volunteers might differ from nonvolunteers in personality make-up and attitudes towards topics such as mental illness and the mentally ill. The questions we sought to answer were as follows: Are volunteers more idealistic, nurturant, aggressive, conforming, etc.? Do they have initially more positive or negative attitudes to the mentally ill? To understand such differences, if they exist, and to relate them to patient outcomes, may help us to know what kinds of individuals should be encouraged to work in this area.

A considerable amount of prior work has been done comparing college student hospital volunteers and nonvolunteers. Knapp and Holzberg (1964) found relatively few personality differences between volunteers and nonvolunteers. Volunteers had higher intraception and nurturance scores and lower change scores on the Edwards Personal Preference Schedule (EPPS) than did

[1] This procedure had originally been used as an "icebreaking" technique in encounter groups.

nonvolunteers, but they did not differ from controls on any of the 10 clinical scales of the Minnesota Multiphasic Personality Inventory (MMPI). In a later study, using a similar sample, Holzberg and Knapp (1965) concluded that volunteers "are not distinctively different from . . . controls in any obvious and demonstrable academic, economic or sociological dimensions [p. 590]." If the Holzberg *et al.* samples are representative of college student volunteers in general, one can conclude that they are quite similar to their nonvolunteer classmates. However, there is need for continued study in this area.

In the present study, a broad range of assessment procedures was used to compare volunteers with nonvolunteers. These included measures used in prior investigations, as well as a number of other personality indices, self-ratings, and specific potential predictor variables, such as, locus of control, social insight, self-disclosure, and philosophy of human nature. Interrelationships among these personality measures were also examined.

Prior research suggests that there are few systematic differences between college volunteers and nonvolunteer peers in initial attitudes toward mental illness or toward the mentally ill (Turner, Holzberg, & Knapp, 1967). Volunteer groups, however, have been shown both by Turner *et al.* (1967), using the Gough Adjective Checklist, and Cowen, Zax, and Laird (1966), using a semantic differential technique, to have more idealistic attitudes than their nonvolunteer peers. This is another area requiring further exploration, and is investigated in the present research.

C. Changes in Volunteer Attitudes

What changes in attitudes toward the mentally ill and mental illness, if any, take place in college students after participation in helping programs for chronic patients? How does participation modify the students' views of mental illness and his awareness of the problems of the total institution? Here, we are concerned with educational and personal values that the program may have for the student. At a time of critical manpower shortages, it is important to ascertain whether a concrete, meaningful exposure to an action-oriented helping program is more effective as a recruiting mechanism for the mental health fields, than lectures, discussions or impassive descriptive materials. The question of change in the volunteer has been accorded a fair amount of prior attention. For example, several studies have reported significant positive change in volunteer attitudes toward self, the mentally ill, and concepts related to mental illness following participation in a human service project. Turner *et al.* (1967) found that after serving in a companionship program, volunteers viewed the "typical mental patient" as more nurturant and more capable of forming meaningful relationships than they did before the program. Cowen *et al.* (1966) found that college volunteers rated emotionally disturbed youngsters more favorably after having participated in an after-school day-care project with them. The same volunteers' evaluations of "elementary schools" as an institutional concept, were less positive after their experience in the program.

Scheibe (1965), reported that volunteers who had participated in a summer project in a mental hospital positively changed their descriptions of the typical mental patient and their self-ratings. Holzberg, Gewirtz, and Ebner (1964), summarizing their findings on student attitude change after participation in human service programs with schizophrenics, reported "changes in the direction of a more realistic understanding of mental illness, [and] more positive attitudes toward the mentally ill [p. 302]." Collectively, these studies highlight positive changes in self-attitudes and in attitudes toward the mentally ill in postprogram evaluations.

In this study, we were also concerned with changes in the volunteers' evaluations of the "mental hospital." Conceivably, student attitudes toward the hospital could become more negative as a result of program participation, since the program inevitably exposes the student to the unfortunate conditions under which the chronic patient lives (see p. 4). Such conditions, well described by other observers of large mental institutions (e.g., Goffman, 1961), readily foster an anti-institutional orientation in outside observers, especially ones who identify closely with the patients and their welfare.

D. Volunteer–Process Relationships

At the outset, we believed that there might be relations between student activities during the group session and patient change, which would help to clarify questions of program effectiveness. It would indicate how an "overall program," with specifiable common denominators, using nonprofessionals as helpers, is differentially operationalized by the activities of a given volunteer and his particular patients. Does it make any difference in terms of patient outcome as to what actually transpires in the group? For example, in terms of beneficial effects on patients, are there differences between heavy group use of active verbal interaction versus passively listening to the radio?

Several additional issues in this area merit comment. In order to examine process-outcome relations, a measure of process that reliably describes the transaction being studied is required. How complex this process is and how much leeway a volunteer-leader has in determining it are subject to constraints. For example, if institutional policy limits patient activities, or if there are space problems or a lack of materials and supplies, certain process interactions and events are functionally limited. Assuming some freedom of decision and leeway in choice of activities, other questions take on importance, as, for example, the relation between volunteer personality and attitude variables and the nature of process interaction with patients. Illustratively, are "quiet" and "outgoing" volunteers different in the way they interact with patients and how they conduct groups?

Two related temporal process questions can also be posed. First, how do the various measures of process change over time? Second, how, in the more global sense, do volunteers perceive the group's function over time? Thus, three classes of process questions have been raised: those pertaining to the measurement of process, its variability, and changes in it over time; antecedent questions dealing with relations between volunteer attributes and process events; and consequent questions dealing with the actual process events as they relate to patient outcomes.

We have long been concerned with process in psychological research. Typically, when new treatment conditions are studied, whether educational, psychotherapeutic, or pharmacological, the initial question asked is "Does the method work?" Once a method is established as workable, focus shifts to a second-level question, "*How* does it work?", a scientifically significant question that implicates the study of component processes. The importance of process-analysis rests on two factors. Though we tend to group methods of treatment conditions under handy overall labels, such conditions are far from homogeneous. What we call psychotherapy, for example, is a mélange of techniques, differentially grouped and applied. There may be relatively little overlap in the actual behaviors, statements, and interventions of the therapists doing intensive psychoanalysis and those doing systematic desensitization. Even within so-called homogeneous "schools," as, for example, client-centered therapy, there are sharp individual differences in technique and implementation. In the last analysis, a method becomes operational through the specific actions and statements of a person who describes himself as a representative of that approach.

Similarly, treatment methods are conglomerates of many things—relational qualities, spoken words, modes of structure, nonverbal aspects of communications, etc. All these tend to be lumped together as *the* approach, or method. If positive patient change occurs, it is difficult to know which of the treatment's complex array of ingredients are active and which are inert. Process analysis, by breaking down complex global units into more discrete components or combinations, helps to identify more and less effective components, and, by focusing on those, to improve the effectiveness of the technique.

A problem in using relatively untrained nonprofessionals in helping programs, is that they are, to a considerable extent, left to their own resources. As has been suggested earlier, there may be value to this because it fosters freedom of exploration. However, it also means that widely divergent behaviors and processes will occur to the extent that the concept of "overall program" has meaning only in terms of broad guidelines and common denominators. Thus, it is important to determine what nonprofessionals actually do in their contacts with patients, and which activities and behaviors, from a broad potential array, are most helpful to patients. This issue has largely been neglected in research on prior programs using nonprofessionals, but its potential for putting this movement on a sounder scientific footing is considerable.

VI. SUMMARY AND OVERVIEW

This volume describes an investigation of the effectiveness of college-student volunteers as interpersonal help-agents with chronic, mental hospital patients. The study is motivated by two facts, both of which create serious current problems for the mental health fields. The first is the ineffectiveness of past and current treatment approaches for major mental illness. Mute living testimony to this ineffectiveness is found in the hundreds of thousands of human beings who spend their lives in the total mental institution. The second problem is the widespread shortage of professional mental health manpower. This situation grows ever more acute both because of the broadening definitional scope of abnormal psychology and the constantly increasing demand for professional services in new settings and for new orders of human problems. Need and demand outstrip resources, meaning that many in need of help cannot be reached. In this unfavorable supply-demand market, mental hospital inmates who are out-of-the mainstream, most readily forgotten, and nonvocal, are especially susceptible to being short-changed.

This project explores the extent to which the goals of more effective treatment for the total psychological casualty, and expansion of the mental health manpower pool, can be simultaneously furthered by a single program—one in which students are used as helping agents with institutional patients experiencing extreme psychological dysfunction. Another basic aim is to study the student volunteers intensively, in terms of how they differ from other college students, how they change as a function of program participation, and which of their qualities relate to positive patient outcomes. As we have pointed out, this study is by no means unique in pursuing these two objectives, either singly or in combination. Its special contribution if any, will be found in the array of research questions it poses about the experimental program, and in the techniques used to examine these questions. We are also keenly aware that the program itself can, at best, be only a partial approach to the vast and complex problem of major mental illness.

A detailed outline of the research design will be presented in Chapter 3, as well as a summary of the studies' major questions and principal findings. A brief overview is provided here to establish a preliminary framework for the materials to follow.

Thirty undergraduates met regularly with small groups of chronic hospitalized patients over a 5½-month period seeking to promote social and verbal interaction. Demographically comparable nontreated controls were included in the study. The students approach to patients was varied, and often novel and imaginative. Patient status was evaluated before and after the program using a comprehensive battery of performance and behavior measures. The findings were complex because not all patients stayed in the program, and change rates were uneven across patient groups. Initially healthier patients were both less likely to remain in the program and less likely to profit from it if they did stay in. Some student–patient combinations (e.g., female student leader and male patients) produced more favorable outcomes than did others. Regardless of outcome, patients expressed more favorable attitudes to college students following the program.

Student group leaders were not strikingly different from nonvolunteer controls in attitude or personality makeup. Following their program activities, students rated patients more favorably and evaluated mental hospitals less favorably than they had before the program. Few of the array of personality and attitude measures taken on student leaders at the start of the program related to effective patient outcomes. One exception was the moderate prediction to effectiveness deriving from qualities such as warmth and understanding judged by peers and observers in a preexperiment behavior rating situation based on actual group interactions.

In the chapters to follow, a detailed account of the objectives of this investigation, its methodology, findings, and implications will be presented. Both the objective research findings and the softer, qualitative, human aspects of the project are considered. Hopefully, in blending these two strands, the reader can achieve a broader perspective and better "feel" for what has actually taken place and for the further steps that are logically indicated.

Chapter 2

THE STATE HOSPITAL: A SLEEPING DRAGON

While the first chapter considered general issues in the care and treatment of chronic hospitalized patients, this chapter focuses on a particular state mental institution, the Rochester State Hospital, site of the present investigation. The authors are keenly aware that the structure, living conditions and policies of that institution markedly influenced the conduct of the project.

I. THE MENTAL HOSPITAL

A. Evolution to the Present: Some Early Dragon Kickers

The history of mental hospitals in the United States is one of exposé and reform on the one hand, and public apathy on the other. Concern for the identified mental patient has been characterized by its cyclicity. Brief periods of exposé and reform of existing conditions have typically been followed by lack of concern and return to earlier unfortunate conditions. The early American moral-treatment philosophy, described by Bockhoven (1963), focused on small group living and the mingling of patients and staff. This forerunner of what is now described as the "therapeutic community" (Jones, 1953) was gradually phased out as European immigration to the United States increased during the mid and late 19th century. The influx of "foreigners" into public hospitals was a major factor contributing to the waning of public concern, and to the advent of public disregard. Ironically, Dorothea Dix's crusade to empty the jails and to fill the mental hospitals helped to change the latter from therapeutic communities to overcrowded custodial hospitals. As her success increased, so did the numbers of mental hospital inmates and, with increasing numbers, came the change from a treatment orientation to a business administration philosophy (Grob, 1966; Greenblatt & Levinson, 1965). By the 1860's, the typical American psychiatric journal was more a business management publication than a clinical or scientific journal. Together with the decline of moral treatment there was a corresponding drop in hospital discharge rates. Thus the accumulation of "chronic patients" in state institutions began.

Clifford Beers' (1921) turn-of-the-century exposé, based on his own experience as a patient in a mental institution, marked the birth of the 20th century mental health movement. Since then, mental hospitals have once again been periodically exposed, reformed and reorganized. Heightened disillusionment with the existing state hospital system arose when the Joint Commission on Mental Health and Illness completed its report in 1961. At that time, the Commission recommended unequivocally that all new state hospitals be limited to 1000 beds or less, and that no patients should be added to state hospitals already having more than 1000 beds. Yet, large state mental hospitals are still very much with us; moreover, they are likely to continue to be. As already suggested, while our most recent thrust in adding new mental health facilities has been to establish community mental health centers, large mental hospitals and the chronic patients they house remain as ever-present problems for the "helping" professions.

Acute as is the general mental health manpower situation, it is magnified manyfold in state hospitals. Society's professional manpower resources in mental health are allocated primarily to outpatient treatment and, to a lesser extent, to inpatient private hospitals. Yet, according to Schofield (1964), "over one-half of all hospital beds in the country are occupied by mental patients, and there are 600,000 psychotic patients housed in public and private mental hospitals at any given time [p. 1]." Albee (1967a) has further noted that, while half of all admissions for mental disorder are to general hospitals, many of these patients are quickly transferred to state institutions when their 30 days of hospital insurance pass. Such institutions, overcrowded with patients, are also understaffed. Of the 300 state hospitals in the United States, 112 have four or fewer staff psychiatrists (Albee, 1967b).

Given the situation we have just described, it is hardly surprising that the typical treatment for chronic patients, who make up the major portion of the state hospital population, consists of drugs, custodial care, or both. The patient has little contact with other human beings, save for his fellow patients. This is due not to staff neglect, but to staff shortage. Gendlin (1966) has called these thousands of patients "people who are abandoned." His comments are relevant:

> Being in a hospital, particularly a state hospital, is a late, visible, physical dramatization of their being disconnected from the world. And this is the disease we try to treat in the hospital! . . . Being isolated in a hospital in physical space is at least the second sense in which . . . [the patient] has been abandoned. First he was abandoned many times in interpersonal space [p. 10].

B. The Rochester State Hospital

The foregoing remarks largely summarize the more detailed account presented in Chapter 1 and describe the hypothetical instance of the large mental hospital. How they apply to the setting for the present project, the Rochester State Hospital, bears consideration!

1. EARLY HISTORY AND DESCRIPTION

The Rochester State Hospital (RSH) is a 3200-bed institution established in 1824 as a county hospital. It was enlarged in 1893, and converted to a state facility in 1891. Its history is not atypical for state mental institutions. Originally built at the edge of the city limits, the hospital is now close to suburban housing developments. Its seven buildings are located on a 292-acre tract. Rochester State serves a six-county area in Central-Western New York. Its patient population is composed largely of lower-income people, and those who lack hospitalization insurance. Patients sent to Rochester State from area private psychiatric facilities are generally viewed by the referring agent as treatment failures.

The four older RSH buildings, erected in the 1930's and segregated by sex, house approximately 2000 patients, half of whom are geriatric patients. Most of these are individuals who have been passed through treatment facilities for more acute problems and are now considered to be "chronic patients." The high proportion of geriatric patients in this setting is consistent with patient censuses in other similar institutions. As the standard of living has advanced, and as medical technology has improved, the proportion of older inmates in mental hospitals has sharply increased; indeed in some ways such settings have become one of society's favored repositories for the elderly.

2. THE HOSPITAL STAFF

The general orientation of the hospital is custodial, particularly in the chronic buildings. Each of the four chronic buildings has one physician whose primary function is to handle the medical problems of its approximately 500 inmates. Management and custodial care are the responsibility of the building supervisor, a nurse who is subordinate to the chief of nursing. Each building supervisor has a staff of nurses and attendants who manage the custodial needs of the unit. At the top of the administrative hierarchy are the hospital superintendent, the clinical director, and the administrative director.

The hospital has a psychology department and a department of social service, but their time is so much taken up by the needs and problems of acutely disturbed patients, particularly children and adolescents, that their ability to become involved in the chronic buildings is minimal.

3. THE STATUS QUO: A SLEEPING DRAGON

The atmosphere in the chronic buildings is one of dimly-lit silence, punctuated by occasional "episodes" from a disturbed patient. The day rooms on each ward are large and empty, sparsely furnished with several wooden chairs and a TV set. A distinct aura of inactivity pervades. The patients sleep in bed-lined dormitories with no storage facilities for private possessions. Although occupational and recreational therapy is offered, few chronic patients attend these activities. The staff is so small and facilities so limited that attendance cannot be encouraged. While a few patients spend time helping the ward personnel in cleaning – there is no janitorial staff – and others have a grounds or city pass or work in the hospital laundry, most spend the day sitting quietly. There are a few "open wards" but most are locked.

As a result of the lack of public and private concern about the well-being of state hospital patients, often expressed through minimal budgets, the nonprofessional staff is both too small and underpaid. Staff efforts necessarily center around physical care and insuring patient conformity to hospital rules. There is a need to keep the wards as quiet and controlled as possible. Regimentation is the style of life. In short, the atmosphere is very much like that described by Goffman (1961) as predisposing to the development of the syndrome of "institutionalism."

C. Changing a Social System: Awakening the Sleeping Dragon

Faced with a situation such as the one described in the previous section, the question is obvious: How can one begin to have meaningful impact on the entrenched social system that is a state hospital? In many ways, the challenge of introducing significant change into a state hospital can be likened to the problem of awakening a sleeping dragon—one on a continuous dose of thorazine! In order to awaken such a dragon, one must learn how it functions and then carefully decide how to go about the task.

1. HOW TO AVOID BEING DEVOURED

In the absence of direct administrative power by the would-be innovators, individual cooperation of key hospital people is necessary. It is never obvious from formal charts of organizational structure, who such key people are. Indeed, the charts often serve only to mislead. In short, one must *learn* the existing social system. The task of finding out and negotiating a system for change is a difficult one.

If the dragon is awakened with a sharp poke in the ribs, he may devour the awakener and go back to sleep, content with having rid himself of annoyance. A more optimistic approach is to awaken the dragon gently with whispered suggestions and some demonstrated success at improving its welfare. Short of revolution, this is the problem in changing any large and entrenched social system: One must introduce new goals or demonstrate that changes will be more effective than present methods for achieving the institution's stated goals—in this case, effective treatment of chronic patients. Graziano (1969) describes in detail his experience in trying to change a community's "mental health establishment." His admonition that "innovators, by definition, introduce change [while] . . . power structures resist change [p. 10]" is relevant to state hospitals as well.

2. THE INTRACTABLE DRAGON

One potential problem of the large, impersonal organizational structure is its tendency to rigidify. As institutions survive their originators, succeeding administrators often perceive maintenance of the institution and its evolved ways of doing things as ends in themselves. In the case of public institutions such as state hospitals, to do so is often detrimental to the welfare of its constituents. For example, if one objective of a state hospital is to rehabilitate patients, it is sensible to develop work programs as a part of the rehabilitation effort. If the institution is also constrained by minimal budgets, it may make sense to have patients work in order to help meet their living expenses. Thus, it is both business-like and humane to assign capable patients to useful work, as, for example, in the hospital laundry, in gardening, etc. Through such programs, patients can both be "rehabilitated," in the sense of performing useful work, and can help to defray heavy hospital expenses.

Unfortunately, over a period of years, the hospital may become dependent on work performed by its inmates. If that happens, hospital administrators may inadvertently assign maintenance a higher functional priority than patient treatment. Thus, if a patient is offered a new treatment program that interferes with his work schedule in an industry that helps to support the hospital, administrators may refuse to allow him to participate in the program. This is especially the case if the treatment is seen to upset hospital routine and to be of as yet unproven value. This danger is greatest for "chronic resident" patients in whom the maintenance role is most likely to be perpetuated. In encouraging such roles, the hospital often abandons the goal of effective patient treatment.

Sanders, Smith, and Weinman (1967) recently considered reasons for resistance to change by large institutions, ranging from established and rigidified organizational structures to professional competition. Add to such considerations, severe manpower shortages and low budgets with consequent low salaries and one can understand why state hospitals maintain entrenched methods and custodial goals. While this is generally so, it is clearest above all for the chronic patient units.

3. ALTERNATIVES TO REVOLUTION

For those who seek to break through the custodial orientation of large mental hospitals, there are at least several prospective alternatives. One obvious way to change the operation and/or goals of a social system is simply to replace its key administrators—a step that is considerably easier to verbalize than to achieve. Alternately, one can try to convince administrators to change policies and practices. The latter is often a "necessary, but insufficient" step. In the case of a system such as Rochester State, for example, while formal lines of power are easily identifiable, actual lines are not. The position of *de facto* power varies across buildings. In one case, it may be a building supervisor (the head nurse), in another, the individual ward nurse, and in a third, the physician. At Rochester State, the central administration has little direct control over the chronic buildings. In order to have hopes of fostering constructive change, one must deal directly with the *de facto* powers in each building. Replacing top administrators in the hospital's organizational chart, which was neither considered, nor possible, in this case, would not necessarily have led to salutary social change. Neither would convincing central administration to institute policy change, without also convincing the *de facto* powers, lead to such change.

4. POWER TO THE NONPROFESSIONAL: THE DRAGON KICKER'S TACTIC

Ellsworth (1968) has suggested that where the nonprofessional hospital staff has power, change can be implemented by increasing communication between the professional and nonprofessional staff, and using nonprofessionals in vital ways as treatment, rather than custodial personnel. Here, the dragon awakener requires considerable administrative power over both the professional and the nonprofessional staff.

Sanders *et al.* (1967) have described two general approaches to changing a hospital's goals in situations where the instigator has little or no power. One is to collaborate with those in power, and the other is to move ahead on one's own resources and attempt to demonstrate both program success and the absence of disaster following innovation. With collaboration, one risks diluting new goals to the point of ineffectiveness. The risk of independent demonstration is that the results will not be convincing, or that they will create antagonism.

At the time this project was first considered, the present investigators were in a uniquely peripheral power position with respect to the institution. The first two authors (J.R. & J.C.) were psychology interns at Rochester State with no administrative power whatsoever. The third author (E.L.C.) was a professor of psychology at a nearby university with minimal contact, and no power at Rochester State Hospital. Given this situation, the authors decided to attempt to modify methods and goals for dealing with chronic patients, through the collaborative path—first, by obtaining central administration's sanction for a small pilot project. Through the hospital's chief psychologist, they presented a plan for the use of college students as potential helping agents with patients. It was proposed that several students be introduced into chronic patient buildings, and that they be left largely to their own devices to work with small groups of patients. While this idea per se was not a new one (as suggested in Chapter 1), such a program had not previously been considered at Rochester State. Indeed, the legal questions and ethical problems encountered during the initial "go-around" seemed insurmountable. Nevertheless, the hospital administration eventually agreed to permit such an intervention, subject to approval by building supervisors. Each supervisor had to be "sold" on the merits of the proposal and reassured about possible program effects on "his" building. Thus, it was necessary to convince building personnel, including nonprofessional staff, not only that the proposed program might be beneficial for patients, but also that it would not disrupt ongoing hospital routine. To do this, a pilot study was conducted prior to the main study. Thus, in a small way, hospital personnel came to see some potential benefit from the unfolding, but still neonatal, program.

The program objective was described during several staff meetings as that of providing chronic patients with a vehicle for small-group social interaction which, if effective, might help to reverse the effects of long-term institutionalization. This was presented in the context of the shortage of personnel on each ward, an omnipresent complaint throughout the hospital, and the opportunity to bring in outside assistance to ease burdens of the regular staff. From the authors' viewpoint, the purposes of the pilot investigation were twofold:

(1) To determine the feasibility of introducing this form of intervention into Rochester State Hospital.

(2) To obtain a preliminary estimate of the effectiveness of college students in this form of treatment.

The immediate consequence of the meetings with building personnel was to arouse suspicion of our motives. The following questions were typical: Were we interested only as "academic researchers?" Did we really care about the patients? Did we think that the staff was not doing its job adequately? A second consequence was to arouse resistance. Once again, high-frequency questions can be cited: Would the program disrupt the ward routine and create more work for the staff? Would "college kids" be able to "handle" mental patients? What about "very disturbed" patients? Would college students be responsible enough to trust in the hospital? Would they obey the rules?

There were at least three concerns underlying these questions:

(1) *Professional jealousy:* College students were seen as bookish adolescents who could not handle the demanding tasks that mental hospital workers had to cope with daily.
(2) *Fear of outsiders:* People who did not "understand" the problems of a mental hospital might make unfair accusations of incompetence. Failings of the staff might thus become public information.
(3) *Creation of additional work:* Disruption of well-established routines might lead to more work for an already overworked staff.

Our strategy at this point was to try to convince ward personnel that they were doing as good a job as possible under trying circumstances and, in fact, were overworked. They were told that the program would in no way evaluate them, but rather would evaluate the students. In full sincerity, we told the staff that no project in the hospital could work well without their cooperation.

Pious abstract words, however, were not enough! Thus, we spent much time simply being in the buildings, small-talking when appropriate, discussing anything that came up, and becoming a familiar and acceptable part of the staff. Thus, a concerted effort was made to change our image from evaluating "foreign bodies" to concerned members of a team, sharing the aim of improving the patient's condition. Although two of the authors were members of the hospital psychology department, housed in the acute treatment building and officially, only marginally related to the chronic wards, we stressed our genuine concern with the latter. At this stage, the hospital Chief of Psychology was most helpful. Over a period of years, he had developed an excellent reputation throughout the hospital and was respected by the staff. His introduction and implicit acceptance of project objectives was frequently enough of an "icebreaker" to allow us to become acquainted with individual staff members. Thus, over a period of time, we became more acceptable figures personally—sufficiently so to go ahead with our pilot study, which we hoped would ease remaining problems through concrete demonstration.

II. THE PILOT PROJECT: THE DRAGON STIRRING

The pilot project proceeded as follows: Two female junior undergraduates, both summer research assistants at the University of Rochester, served as student leaders. Neither had any prior experience with mental patients and their participation was voluntary, independent of their assigned duties. Twenty-four female patients were selected from the files of the four chronic buildings as subjects for the pilot study. Their mean length of hospitalization was 10 years (range 1–25). Most were diagnosed as chronic schizophrenics. The 24 patients were divided into three groups of eight, matched for age, length of hospitalization, diagnosis (paranoid or nonparanoid), marital status, and race. Each volunteer met with one of the two eight-patient experimental groups twice weekly over 4 weeks, for a total of eight group meetings. The third, a control group, continued its usual hospital routine without intervention.

The volunteers were given neither specific instructions nor constraints about what they should do in their group meetings; rather, they were left to their own ingenuity. The only guideline given was that they should try to foster group interaction. The activities of the pilot groups varied from bingo to singing, talking, and playing games.

Within the two weeks before the summer pilot program started, and again at its conclusion, all 24 patients were individually tested on five measures sampling the dimensions of psychomotor, perceptual-motor, and verbal functioning. Detailed descriptions of the measures and the results of this pilot study have been reported elsewhere (Rappaport & Chinsky, 1968). Of importance here are two general observations: Despite only eight sessions, restricted to a 1-month period, and with a very small N (16 experimental subjects) the volunteers appeared to have had beneficial impact upon these chronic patients. Perhaps even more important, their involvement was accepted by the hospital and proved to be administratively feasible.

Somewhat to the authors' surprise, the students were well accepted by regular hospital staff. They got along well in informal interactions with staff members and demonstrated that they were responsible people. None of the feared negative "incidents" occurred; in fact, patients reported that they enjoyed group meetings. The students neither questioned the staff's ability nor created more work for staff. On occasions, they even helped them! Thus, demonstrating the program through the summer pilot project allayed anxieties and reduced resistance to the major project.

A. Student Attitude

The students' involvement with "their" patients was gratifying—a harbinger of the kinds of relationships that were later to develop during the main experimental project. For example, one of the undergraduate leaders met with her group in a basement room from 1:00 to 2:00 p.m. on a hot July afternoon. As the meeting ended, she and her eight patients entered the elevator to return to the second floor wards. The elevator stopped on the first floor and the second volunteer entered with her group of eight patients. The students had never seen each other's patient group. They traveled together, in silence, to the second floor. Later that week, one author, acting as supervisor and consultant, met with the first student leader to discuss group contacts. She described the elevator encounter, and with great relief and pride said that she was ". . . so happy about my patients . . . they look so much better; they seem so much more alive and interesting than [X's] group." The second student met independently with another author for her supervision session and also told with pride of the elevator encounter. She was pleased that *her* patients looked and acted so much better than the first group! It was only a few days later when the two authors discussed the supervision sessions that they realized what had happened. When all four of us next met, we understood a little better than before, what human relationships are. We were to see this many times in the next months.

B. Hospital Attitudes: A Passive Dragon?

The positive summer experience produced sufficient data and enough of an advance in acceptance to win agreement from hospital staff that the program should be continued and expanded—even to the point of including patients working in the laundry. Staff in three of the four chronic buildings were now willing to have the new program take place, although they did not wish to help run it.

1. BUILDING D: A NUMB LEG

Supervisors in the fourth building (Building D) refused, functionally, to participate, though they did not say so directly. Since central administration had authorized—indeed approved—the intervention, staff in Building D was unable, out-and-out, to reject the program; instead it utilized *de facto* powers to deflect it. Thus, system-change in Building D was resisted even when its sister buildings accepted it, most probably because the physician in charge was very much concerned about autonomous administrative control in her unit. She and the nursing supervisor had developed, over a period of years, an effective relationship free of the "outside" control represented by central hospital administration.

A simple "factual-scientific" chronicle of the summer pilot project fails substantially to convey significant qualitative and atmospheric elements of the experience. Before the preliminary experiment could take place, two essential steps had to be carried out in each of the buildings. First, we had to become known to, and trusted by, nonprofessional ward personnel, and second, we had to develop access to patient records in order to select a patient sample that met the overall requirements of the research design. The obstacles and misfortunes attendant with these seemingly simple, straightforward steps were legion. Only the salving effects of time and distance put these experiences in a type of tragicomic relief; at the time they elicited precious few responses other than those of frustration and anger.

In the following paragraphs, we shall present several of our experiences as they relate to the fruitless attempt to initiate the program in Building D.

Access to the wards in each of the buildings in question required a different key from the ones the authors carried for their prime assignment on the acute treatment unit. Issuance of such keys for "outsiders" was in violation of existing hospital regulations for these wards. Thus, for access to, and egress from, the wards, we had to be let in and out directly by the ward supervisor. Since the supervisor of Building D proved to be an extraordinarily busy person, merely to enter or leave the ward took on the quality of a superhuman effort. On the few occasions when she did allow us to enter the ward, she remained very close to us, stating as her reason for this ". . . men might upset the female patients." This same explanation was also given as a further reason why keys could not be issued. Accordingly, we found it extremely difficult to obtain basic patient information or to relate, with any freedom whatever, to the nonprofessional ward staff.

Since patient records were housed in the supervisor's office, it was also necessary to obtain her direct authorization to look at these. The authors' research assistants were denied access to the records on grounds of their confidentiality. The authors themselves were permitted access only during specified and restricted times. Staff meetings in the mornings conflicted with most of those times. The hours from 11:00 a.m. to 12:00 noon were deemed permissible, but the office needed to be locked during the lunch hour. The supervisor's rounds from 1:00 to 3:00 p.m. eliminated early afternoons, and 3:00 to 5:00 p.m. was a "bad time." Evenings were out of the question.

A further, severe "body-blow" came when we were told that no rooms were available for use by student-patient groups. Thus the program was effectively eliminated in one of the four chronic buildings. We decided that a three-legged limping dragon was better than a sleeping one, and proceeded in the other buildings.

C. Value of the Pilot Study: Training the Dragon

The pilot study was an invaluable experience, both for the hospital and the authors. Not only were we able to try out the group-meeting format and specific research evaluation tools, but were also able to circumvent administrative difficulties in the main study, based on the experiences of the summer project and the knowhow derived therefrom. More importantly, as the hospital personnel became accustomed to us and to the project, resistance decreased. Though somewhat shaken, we were also a bit wiser and ready for the main study.

It was then that we reached our next administrative hurdle. Discussion and observation had suggested that the best times for small group meetings in the main study would be in the early evenings between 6:00 and 8:30 p.m. This was the time of day when patients were most often alone, with no visitors, no activities, and no work on the ward. This was also the time when the staff-to-patient ratio was at its lowest. Frequently, only one attendant was on duty for a ward housing as many as 70 inmates. Though the 6:00–8:30-p.m. meeting time offered several prospective advantages, it also created problems. For example, in order to transport patients to the group meetings held in small rooms off the ward, the night staff member would have to leave the ward unattended. The students could not assemble patients themselves because they were not permitted to have keys. The only solution seemed to be to allow volunteer attendants assigned to the project to work overtime.

Here was the first acid test of active support from the central administration. Its initial response was that the hospital could not afford this additional expense. Accordingly, during the first several weeks of the program, the authors assembled the patients—more than 125 on each of two nights. We had decided to begin the project with a single evening meeting per group, per week, and, in order to have enough rooms for the available meeting-times, one group of student leaders met with patient groups on Monday 6:00 to 7:00 p.m., another 7:20 to 8:20 p.m., and two others on Tuesday, beginning in early November. By February, when the project was to move into full gear, we expected to increase the frequency of meetings from one to two nights weekly, which would mean two Monday—Wednesday and two Tuesday—Thursday student groups. Given the responsibilities of project administration, research, consultation, student supervision, and hospital liaison, it was clear that we would be unable to assemble the patients ourselves four nights a week. The realities of this situation were presented to the hospital superintendent, coupled with a supporting appeal for additional help from the Chief Psychologist. This led to an agreement which allowed ward attendants to work evening overtime hours in support of the project. An initial indication of change in Rochester State Hospital policy had been achieved. For the first time, the hospital took an active rather than a passive stance with respect to the program. We were to wait several months before further active support was given, but at the time, the approximately $90.00 per week in overtime money spent on treatment for some 256 patients, represented a faintly blinking eye in an awakening dragon.

III. CHANGING THE UNIVERSITY'S SOCIAL SYSTEM

A second important problem, admittedly less complex, was being dealt with in parallel. If large numbers of patients were to be provided with a meaningful human-contact experience, then substantial numbers of helpers would have to be identified and recruited. For reasons considered in the preceding chapter, it seemed logical to suppose that program-staffing needs could be met through the prospectively sizable pool of college undergraduates available at the University of Rochester. A principal need, however, was to find a regularizing mechanism for this, which gave promise of simultaneously rendering effective patient service and fulfilling the educational and personal goals of students.

A. Undergraduates: The Need for Relevance

Over a period of several years, it had become apparent that undergraduates at the University of Rochester had a growing interest in human-service activities. Indeed, several *ad hoc* human service programs, involving small numbers of students working for short periods of time, had been conducted both in a mental hospital (Klein & Zax, 1965) and a school setting (Cowen, Zax, & Laird, 1966). As these activities became better known, the demand for such participation by students increased. Thus, at the time the present program was conceived, as would still be true today, one could clearly detect among students a strongly felt need to become involved in experiences that bridged the gap between the academic ivory-tower and existing, entirely real problems of society and of the surrounding community. The proposed project seemed to have that type of potential.

B. Psychology 278

In the summer of 1967, a proposal was formulated to develop a community-service experience for students, for academic course credit—a prospectively constructive broadening of the psychology department's and the University's network of educational offerings. Through the third author, then serving as Director of Clinical Training in the department of psychology, a prospectus was submitted for a new undergraduate offering, Psychology 278: "Seminar and Practicum in Community Mental Health." The course was approved by the appropriate university curriculum committee and by the university faculty, and thus became the formal vehicle by which undergraduates were recruited for this project as group leaders to work with chronic, hospitalized mental patients.

As a small footnote to this process, it should be noted that the request was also made that the new course be graded as pass–fail. This seemed desirable in that the major criterion for evaluation of a student's performance was change in patient status. This variable is realistically constrained by factors such as the patient's initial status, program limits, hospital regulations and policies, student personality, interaction of student personality with patient personality, and the nature of patient disorder. Since none of the latter factors is within the student's "control," patient outcome was not readily subject to the traditional college grading system. The hope was that the pass–fail system could be invoked with a fail grade to be given primarily in the case of gross derelection of clinical responsibility. The request for the pass–fail grading system was denied. In the end, students were asked to do several papers in areas of their interest, and grades for the course were assigned on the basis of their segmented intellectual effort as reflected in these assigned exercises, independent of their clinical activity with patients which was at the very core of the experience. Three years later, the course remains a central and popular one in the department's undergraduate curriculum. The struggle to convert its grading system to a straight pass–fail continued, and has only recently won acceptance.

C. Recruiting Students

With Psychology 278 established, during the summer of 1967 a preliminary announcement was drawn-up, in the form of a letter to the 150 junior and senior psychology majors of record at the University of Rochester, describing the prospective "278" sequence in general terms (Figure 2.1). It was stated that the course would combine seminar-discussion and practicum aspects, largely in a step-sequence. In addition, several prospective practicum assignments, including the Rochester State Hospital program, were identified. Of the 150 letters sent out, approximately 50% were returned indicating a desire to register for such a course in the fall. Those expressing interest were advised that a screening interview would be required some time during the two-day period immediately preceding fall registration.

Prospective course candidates were interviewed briefly before classes started in the fall in an effort to form some judgment of the seriousness of their motivation and, hopefully, to screen out manifestly upset students or those who might become unduly troubled through personal contact with patients in distress. The emphasis was on gross negative screening rather than trying to pick "stars." During the interview, students were advised about the prospective range of clinical activities, the need for a totally serious commitment, the amount of time that would be required (up to 8 hours per week), and the heavy collection of research data, both for themselves and their "assigned patients," from start to finish of the program. Application of screening criteria eliminated several students; several others decided not to take the course because of the nature or magnitude of the requirements, and still others were unable to register because of schedule conflicts.

Forty-eight students, 24 men and 24 women, were accepted on a full year basis. Thirty-two of these, 16 men and 16 women, were assigned to the Rochester State Hospital program; the remaining 16 were assigned to an after-school companionship and activity program with primary graders in Rochester's public schools, described elsewhere (Cowen, Carlisle, & Kaufman, 1969). In the main, these assignments were based on expressed student preference. Actually, there were more applicants for the course than could be accommodated, including several nonpsychology majors who learned of it by word of mouth. Additional latecomers sought to enroll during the first weeks of the semester and some 20 others asked permission to join the program for the second semester. These facts imply strong interest in and receptivity for this type of undergraduate experience.

D. Design of the Course

The initial 10 weeks of the course were devoted to aspects of the field of community mental health, beginning with a brief history of the mental health movement, its origins and pattern of evolution, as well as current unresolved problems and issues. Alternative conceptual models, including particularly the medical and preventive models, were reviewed with special emphasis on their underlying assumptions and implementing practices. Detailed consideration was given to issues and problems in three broad areas: (1) demands, needs, manpower and resources in the mental health fields; (2) the limitations of traditional and existing approaches (e.g., psychotherapy, and large mental hospitals); and (3) mental health services for the poor. A second round of meetings sought to describe emergent, innovative programs designed to provide solutions to pressing problems in these same three areas. New uses of a variety of nonprofessionals in many different settings, including mental hospitals, were considered, as were alternative approaches to psychotherapy and new mental health programs for the poor.

The text for the course was Cowen, Gardner, and Zax (1967). For each subarea, required and recommended readings were given, including journal articles, book chapters, and entire volumes (see Table 2.1). Examples of the latter included: Albee (1959), Goffman (1961), Harrington (1962), Schofield (1964), and Riessman, Cohen, and Pearl (1964).

The "lecture-discussion" portion of the course generated considerable and sometimes heated participation. The prevailing bias of the instructors was

Figure 2.1. Letter inviting students to register for the practicum course.

Dear Student:

There is a rapidly growing demand for human services in the mental health areas combined with a realization that the number of existing professional persons are unable to meet the demand. In an effort to cope with this problem, there has been an increased use of nonprofessional manpower in human services to individuals with emotional difficulties. One source of such manpower is the university undergraduate. Programs utilizing students have been enthusiastically received at places such as Harvard, Wesleyan, and up until now, to a more limited extent, here at the University of Rochester.

The Department of Psychology is planning an extension of programs in this area for the academic year 1967-1968 through the medium of a newly created combined didactic-practicum course, which is to be held for the first time. This course (Psychology 278) will provide an exposure to relevant theory as well as practical experience in the area of community mental health. The course is designed to allow the student to obtain a further understanding of contemporary mental health problems and issues by actually participating in one of several on-going service and research projects.

The experience will consist of three broad components:

1. An orientation to the area of community mental health theory and practice including such issues as manpower problems, the use of nonprofessionals, new treatment approaches, relations to existing mental health professions.
2. Actual practicum experience in a mental hospital, elementary school, and/or a settlement house.
3. On-going supervision and small group discussions with advanced graduate students and faculty.

There will be no formal <u>course</u> requirements for admission; however, a brief initial interview will be necessary. Qualified applicants will be given a battery of psychological tests, <u>following</u> their acceptance into the course. These tests will be used <u>only</u> for research purposes, and will in no way influence acceptance or grades. The point, however, is that all students enrolled in the course will participate in the research aspects of the experience throughout. Grades for the course will be on a pass-fail basis and there will be no exams. Commitment to the course <u>must</u> be made for the full year. It may be possible to work this out on a 0, 4 or 8 credit basis, but the concept of full commitment by all participating students is essential. Participation is didactic and practicum aspects of the course will be variable during the year. It is improbable that the practicum components of the experience will extend over a period of more than five months. During that period, however, actual involvement is likely to total to approximately 5-8 hours per week.

Because of the nature of the course, only a limited number of students can be accepted. Consequently, it is important that you return the enclosed questionnaire so that those who are interested may be scheduled for an interview early in September. Whether or not you are interested in enrolling in this course, we would appreciate it if you would furnish the information requested on the attached sheet and return it in the enclosed stamped envelope.

Please provide the information requested below whether or not you wish to take the course.

NAME____________________CLASS________________

ADDRESS______________________________

HOME________________

____

____

CAMPUS________________

____

1. I would like to enroll in the course for 1967-8 (If answer to question is "yes," do not answer other questions). ____/____ yes no

2. I would like to enroll in the course for 1967-8 but cannot because of prior course commitments or scheduling problems. ____/____ yes no
   (For Juniors or Sophomores - If answer to number 2 is yes, would you like to participate next year?). ____/____ yes no

3. I do not wish to participate in the course ____/____ yes no

   Please give reason:

   I'm not interested in the area

   Course doesn't sound worthwhile

   Other things are more appealing

   Sounds like it would take too much time

   Other (please state)____________________

that there are sharp limitations in the existing mental health order and these shortcomings may be reduced by the varied use of nonprofessionals. The students were concerned about their own lack of credentials and "knowhow" and were skeptical that attributes such as interest, commitment, high level of motivation and enthusiasm, which they accepted as *their* "trump cards," could have meaningful, positive impact on distressed individuals. Students' interest and reactivity was highest not when problems and issues were being delineated abstractly, but rather when concrete programs involving nonprofessionals were considered. Similarly, students expressed a strong need to be armed with technique (an "ersatz" therapist's tool-kit) that would maximize the likelihood of their being able to help others.

TABLE 2.1 *Psychology 278: Seminar–Practicum in Community Mental Health; Readings and 10-Week Course Outline (September, 1967)*

Books and Papers

Albee, G. W. *Mental health manpower trends.* New York: Basic Books, 1959.

Albee, G. W. American psychology in the sixties. *American Psychologist,* 1963 **18,** 90-95.

Caplan, G. *Principles of preventive psychiatry.* New York: Basic Books, 1964.

Cowen, E. L., Gardner, E. A., & Zax, M. (Eds.) *Emergent approaches to mental health problems.* New York: Appleton, 1967. [Course text]

Eysenck, H. J. The effects of psychotherapy: An evaluation. *Journal of Consulting Psychology,* 1952, **16,** 319-324.

Eysenck, H. J. The effects of psychotherapy: A reply. *Journal of Abnormal & Social Psychology,* 1955, **50,** 147-148.

Gans, H. A survey of working and lower class studies. In F. Riessman, J. Cohen, & A. Pearl (Eds.) *Mental health of the poor.* New York: Free Press, 1964.

Greenblatt, M. & Levenson, D. J. Mental hospitals. In B. B. Wolman (Ed.) *Handbook of clinical psychology.* New York: McGraw-Hill, 1965.

Goffman, E. *Asylums.* Garden City, New York: Anchor, 1962.

Haggstrom, W. C. The power of the poor. In F. Riessman, J; Cohen, & A. Pearl (Eds.) *Mental health of the poor.* New York: Free Press, 1964.

Harrington, M. *The other America: Poverty in the United States.* Baltimore: Penguin, 1962.

Joint Commission for Mental Health & Illness. *Action for mental health,* New York: Basic Books, 1961.

Poser, E. G. The effect of therapists' training on group therapeutic outcome. *Journal of Consulting Psychology,* 1966, **30,** 283-289.

Rioch, M. J. Changing concepts in the training of therapists.*Journal of Consulting Psychology,* 1966, **30,** 290-292.

Rosenbaum, M. Some comments on the use of untrained therapists. *Journal of Consulting Psychology,* 1966, **30,** 292-294.

Rosenzweig, S. A transvaluation of psychotherapy: A reply to Hans Eysenck. *Journal of Abnormal & Social Psychology,* 1955, **50,** 147-148.

Rosenzweig, S. Calumet. *Journal of Abnormal & Social Psychology,* 1955, **50,** 148.

Sanford, N. The prevention of mental illness. In B. B. Wolman (Ed.) *Handbook of clinical psychology,* New York: McGraw-Hill, 1965.

Sarason, S. B., Levine, M., Goldenberg, I., Cherlin, D. L., & Bennett, E. M. *Psychology in community settings,* New York: Wiley, 1966.

Schofield, W. *Psychotherapy: The purchase of friendship.* Englewood Cliffs, New Jersey: Prentice-Hall, 1964.

Umbarger, C. C., Dalsimer, J. S., Morrison, A. P., & Breggin, P. R. *College students in a mental hospital:* New York: Grune & Stratton, 1962.

Wolpe, J. The comparative clinical status of conditioning therapies and psychoanalysis. In J. Wolpe, A. Salter, & L. J. Reyna (Eds.) *The conditioning therapies.* New York: Holt, 1964.

Course Outline

Unit I: *History & introduction to the field; delineation of issues & problems.*

Reading assignments: Cowen *et al.* Chapter 1
Caplan, Chapters 1, 2
Joint Commission Report Summary
Sanford
Sarason pp. 1-17; 645-649.

Unit II: *Conceptual approaches.*

Reading assignments: Cowen *et al.* Chapters 2, 4.
Schofield.

Unit III: *Detailed consideration of issues and problems.*

A. Demands, needs; manpower and resources.

Reading assignments: Albee, 1959; 1963
Schofield.

B. Effectiveness of existing approaches.

Reading assignments: Greenblatt & Levinson
Eysenck, 1952; 1955
Rosenzweig, 1954, 1955.

C. Mental Health services for the poor.

Reading assignments: Gans
Harrington.

Unit IV: *Emerging resolutions to mental health problems.*

A. Manpower & resources.

Reading assignments: Cowen *et al.* Chapters 6, 7, 12, 19, 20.
Umbarger *et al.*

B. New treatment approaches.

Reading assignments: Cowen *et al.* Chapter 8
Poser
Rioch
Rosenbaum
Wolpe.

C. New ways with the poor.

Reading assignments: Cowen *et al.* Chapters 9, 10, 11.
Haggstrom

Unit V: *Summary.*

Reading assignment: Cowen *et al.* Chapter 21.

As the didactic segments of the course proceeded, specific arrangements for beginning practicum work were finalized. The start of practicum activities dovetailed with completion of the didactic portions of the course. There was a formal transition period during which students visited the hospital, met with key personnel, and were given background about the organizational structure and rules of the hospital and information about patients with whom they were to be working. For the remainder of the academic year, students assigned to Rochester State carried out their practicum assignment, under supervision, as discussed in a later chapter.

Thus, by the start of the academic year 1967–1968, following a summer of negotiating the social systems of both the local state hospital and the university, an innovative program was ready to begin. A major aim, in addition to improved patient service and broader student education, was to evaluate the effects of this program experimentally.

Chapter 3

AN OVERVIEW

This chapter is intended as a capsule summary of the entire investigation, to provide the reader with an overview of its most salient aspects. Since the purposes of the project were considered in detail in Chapters 1 and 2, we begin with a description of the research design, go on to identify the specific student and patient samples, and report on the instruments and techniques used in the evaluation. Finally, we cite the specific questions that the investigation set out to explore and, for each, present a brief resumé of the findings. In that sense, it is proper to regard the chapter as a before-the-fact summary. While the remainder of the volume will, hopefully, add important detail and richness to the report, the project's essential profile and findings are found in this chapter.

I. DESIGN OF THE STUDY

A. Students

Most of the 32 college-student volunteers, all juniors or seniors (mean age, 20–21), were advanced psychology majors and all had some prior academic background in psychology.

At the end of the 10-week didactic portion of the course, described in the preceding chapter, each student was assigned as a group leader to eight chronic schizophrenic patients. In their first 2 months of clinical activity, students met once weekly for 1 hour, with patient groups; thereafter, for the 5½-month duration of the program there were two 1-hour meetings per week. The orientation of the students was to foster patient group interaction. Groups of eight student leaders also met regularly, once a week, with one of the authors, for discussion and supervision. The supervisory meetings were not designed as teaching sessions, but rather as idea-exchanging and problem-centered discussion groups. While the authors were sometimes able to help students to reduce anxiety around a particular problem, the meetings served more to consider issues of program administration and conduct, to communicate and to share information, and to discuss concrete problems of patient handling and their potential resolutions. The content of the meetings ranged broadly and included airings of satisfactions and frustrations experienced by the students in their work, considering how to engage patients and to interact with them; discussing "refractory" patients and special techniques for "handling" them, evaluating the program both from the standpoint of patients and group leaders, and routine administrative matters. A more detailed clinical description of aspects of the group meetings is presented in Chapter 7.

Throughout the program, two of the authors were full-time interns on the psychology staff of the hospital. Their functions included explaining the program to the professional and nonprofessional staff of the hospital, fostering a climate of receptivity for the program, which, in this setting, was both novel and potentially threatening, serving in an administrative–liaison capacity between hospital staff and participating students, reporting on program progress and difficulties, and improving the effectiveness of its operation.

Their carving out of, and immersion in, a largely consultative resource role vis-á-vis college student volunteers constituted a paradigmatic representation of the "mental health quarterback" role that has increasingly come to characterize the day-to-day function of many professionals with respect to nonprofessionals in various clinical settings (Cowen, 1967).

B. Patients

Patients were drawn from three chronic hospital buildings available to the project, each characterized, for many years, by a stable custodial orientation. A total of 256 patients, including an equal number of males and females, constituted the experimental sample for the study. The 32 experimental groups were closely matched for age, education, marital status, length of hospitalization, and psychiatric diagnosis (paranoid versus nonparanoid). The total experimental group was closely matched to a control group of 64 patients, 32 male and 32 female, drawn from the same wards. The overall design of the study is graphically depicted in Table 3.1. A more detailed description of the patient sample is presented in Chapter 4.

TABLE 3.1 *Experimental Design Indicating Number and Sex of Patients and Student Leaders Assigned to Each Cell*

Male patients	Female patients	Totals
	E-Group (male student leaders)	
Student leaders $N = 8$ Patients $N = 64$	Student leaders $N = 8$ Patients $N = 64$	16 Male student leaders 128 Patients in 16 groups
	E-Group (female student leaders)	
Student leaders $N = 8$ Patients $N = 64$	Student leaders $N = 8$ Patients $N = 64$	16 Female student leaders 128 Patients in 16 groups
	C-Group (no student leaders)	
Patients $N = 32$	Patients $N = 32$	64 Patients
	Totals	
160 Male patients	160 Female patients	32 Student leaders } Grand 320 Patients } total

II. EVALUATION

Evaluation of both the patients and student leaders took place before, during, and after the program.

A. Patients

Several weeks before the start of the program, each patient was individually evaluated using a comprehensive test battery. The component assessment procedures were selected in terms of several criteria: sufficient simplicity so that chronic schizophrenics could respond to them; demonstrated ability to discriminate between normals and schizophrenics; and the development of a total test array reflecting a broad spectrum of functions. The final battery included perceptual, cognitive, and psychomotor tests spanning diverse performance functions. To complement these indices, ward behavior ratings were submitted by hospital staff members and group behavior ratings were made by the student leaders. In all, 22 principal measures were used as patient evaluation indices. Additionally, patient attitudes and expectations about college students were evaluated prior to, and at the conclusion of the project. Tests administered directly to patients required, on the average, about 45 minutes. However, because some patients were unable to respond to certain tests, it was necessary to test more than 320 patients to establish the final E and C groups.

During the final 2 weeks of the program, the entire test battery was readministered, again individually, to all patients. Behavior ratings from ward and student judges were also obtained at the "post"-point. Differences between preprogram and postprogram scores on performance tests and rating measures constituted the prime criteria for evaluating patient change as a function of program participation.

B. Students

Student volunteers were evaluated on a number of attitude and personality indices including measures of social insight, self-concept, therapeutic style, locus of orientation, and self-disclosure. In addition, observation of structured, live interactions among small groups of students provided a basis for "before-the-fact" behavioral ratings by peers and supervisors. Each student underwent about 10 hours of assessment before the program began, yielding some 85 measures per student. A portion of this testing, pertaining particularly to attitude measures, was repeated twice for all students, including once at the very end of the program.

Two student-control-groups were included in the study. The first was to determine whether there were differences between students who volunteered for the project and those who did not. The second served as a basis for evaluating change in students' attitudes as a result of having participated in the program.

C. Process Data

Records of student–patient interactions were kept. These included periodic summaries and checklists describing, by category, the nature of student–patient interactions, the frequency of occurrence of these activities, and changes in frequency over time. Each student also kept a log of his impressions, describing events in his group and his reactions to those events. Finally, each student tape-recorded one or more group sessions. These recordings were submitted to judges for rating along relevant interaction dimensions.

Our interest in the process measures was threefold:

(1) to represent, as accurately as possible, the nature of the student–patient transaction;
(2) to determine the relation, if any, between student attitude and personality measures and what actually took place during the group meetings;
(3) to assess relations between what took place in the groups and patient change.

III. MAJOR QUESTIONS AND FINDINGS

The investigation required substantial and, at times, painstaking data collection. In all, there were 256 E-patient *S*s and 64 C-patient *S*s, a total of 320 patient *S*s. In addition, there were 32 student group-leaders (Es) and 91 student controls (Cs). Including both pre- and postevaluations, the study entailed perhaps 1000 hours of subject-testing and assessment, exclusive of the actual patient group sessions and their related process measures. The data obtained permitted us to examine a series of significant questions, several of which have already been identified. For purposes of systematization, however, a brief summary of the salient experimental questions and of the principal findings relevant to each, is presented as follows.

1. How effective is this type of intervention?

This question was approached by comparing the E group, and various of its subcombinations, with the C group in terms of change on the component behavioral and performance measures. Evidence is presented (Chapter 5) to indicate that there were positive changes for the E group in contrast to C. In particular, one subgroup, male patients seen by female students, showed the greatest improvement.

2. What are the demographic and test characteristics of patients who improved most through participation in the program?

In general, demographic characteristics such as age, diagnosis, and marital status failed to predict to outcome. However, pretest measures of patients in the E group predicted reasonably well to outcome, according to the formula that initially *poorer* functioning patients improved the *most.*

3. What attributes characterize patients who "stay" in the program as opposed to those who either leave or become "spotty" attenders?

Once again, it was found that initially *poorer* functioning patients remained closer to the program and attended more regularly than did relatively more intact patients.

4. What changes in patient attitudes occurred as a result of their participation in the program?

Patients developed demonstrably more favorable attitudes toward college students during the program, both absolutely as well in relation to professional caregivers.

5. What differences are there between students who volunteer for the program and those who do not?

In the main, there were few personality or attitude differences between the student volunteers and the nonvolunteer controls.

6. *What changes occur in students as a function of participation in the program?*

In comparison to controls, student leaders developed significantly more positive attitudes toward patients and significantly less favorable attitudes toward the institutional concept of the "mental hospital," following program participation.

7. *What relations are there between student attitude, personality, and behavioral qualities and patient change indices?*

Attitude and personality attributes of students, as measured by standardized tests, predicted poorly to positiveness of patient outcome; however, the actual, observed, *behavioral* qualities of warmth and understanding in student leaders yielded low-level prediction to successful patient outcome.

8. *How did students evaluate their own experience and change in their patient groups?*

A variety of student attitudes toward the program were encountered, but overall, these were quite positive. In some instances, the program experience became an important factor in orienting students toward professional careers in the mental health field. Students clearly perceived considerable patient improvement in group behavior over the course of the program. It was less clear, however, that observed patient improvement was maintained when they returned to the ward setting.

9. *What relationships are there between group process measures and outcome indices?*

Patient groups characterized by a high *talking* ratio tended to have more favorable outcomes. Conversely, those that had high *listening* rates including passive activities such as listening to the radio, TV, and poetry, had less favorable outcomes.

The foregoing is the core series of questions addressed by the project, for which data are available. A number of other less central, largely empirical, questions have also been studied. Additionally, recommendations about the future use of college students in similar settings are offered.

A description of the patients, the students, and our evaluation techniques is presented in Chapter 4. Detailed findings of the study are presented in Chapters 5 and 6 for the patients and college students, respectively. This is done largely as a descriptive narrative, so that the account can be followed in relatively unbroken form. Descriptive reports of our findings, however, are based on supporting statistical analyses of data. Statistical analyses used run the gamut from chi-squares and other nonparametric techniques to correlational methods, to small-sample techniques, *t* ratios, and analyses of variance, through discriminant function analysis and factor analysis. Hopefully, the format adopted will simultaneously serve the needs of those interested primarily in a verbal description of what happened and those with stronger concerns about the scientific base of the investigation.

Chapter 4

PATIENTS, PROCESS, AND STUDENTS

I. PATIENTS AND PATIENT EVALUATION

The patient sample was drawn from three of the four "chronic" buildings at Rochester State, one housing females and two, males. Criteria for including patients in the final sample were fourfold:

(1) Age range, 21–59 years.
(2) Primary diagnosis neither organic nor mental retardate. Most patients were diagnosed "chronic schizophrenic."
(3) Hospitalization at Rochester State continuously for at least 12 months (no upper limit), immediately prior to the start of the study.
(4) Not currently in any form of treatment other than somatic. Most patients were receiving drugs.

Of the potential pool of about 1500 subjects (*S*s) from the three buildings, approximately 70% were excluded because they failed to meet one or more of the above criteria—most often age. Approximately 400 patients who met all criteria were identified from the file survey. Three hundred and twenty who were sufficiently intact to complete testing (e.g., not hallucinating so extensively as to be unable to respond) were selected to participate in the program. The final sample included about 90% of the Rochester State patients who met the fourfold criteria, and within that subset, virtually 100% of those who were testable.

A. Assignment to Groups

The following demographic data were obtained from the files for each patient: age, length of hospitalization, level of education, marital status, race, religion, and diagnosis (paranoid or nonparanoid). The classification paranoid–nonparanoid was made by the first two authors, based on the presence or absence of indicants of delusions in the patients' record. Rather than using "psychiatric diagnosis" as the basis for matching patient groups, the decision was made to do so in terms of the above measures of "social competence" (Zigler & Phillips, 1961a,b,c).

Forty, eight-patient groups (20 male and 20 female) were matched on the above-mentioned variables. Thirty-two of the 40 groups (16 male and 16 female) were randomly assigned to the experimental (E) condition, and eight hypothetical groups, two each from the two male buildings and four from the female building, were assigned to the control (C) condition. Thus, assignment to an eight-patient group was based on a matching procedure using demographic variables, followed by random assignment of the groups, within each building, to the E or C condition. Tables 4.1 A and B present descriptive data for the 40 patient-groups, total males, total females, total E, and total C in terms of the five matching variables. The E and C groups were virtually identical on all demographic variables within sex. Male patients tended to have been hospitalized slightly longer (about 2 years) than females, primarily due to one male building where the average length of hospitalization was about 3 years more than in the other male building. The mean age for all patient groups was 46.99 with subgroup ranges from 46.00 to 49.25. Mean length of hospitalization ranged from 12.01 to 16.85 years for individual groups, with an overall mean of 13.17 years. Female groups had, on the average, two more married members than male groups. The average educational level for individual subgroups was between 8 and 11 years of schooling, and in each group either four or five of its members were diagnosed as paranoid.

In addition to the demographic measures already described, two patients in each group were randomly selected to take the Peabody Picture Vocabulary IQ Test (Dunn, 1959) in order to estimate IQ for the demographic analyses.

In summary, a very careful matching was obtained among the 40 patient-groups, and between the E and C conditions with respect to five basic demographic–descriptive variables widely used in research with schizophrenic patients. This matching procedure closely followed guidelines presented elsewhere for experimental design in research with chronic hospitalized mental patients (e.g., Kandel & Williams, 1964; Fairweather, 1967). Because of the representativeness of the selected matching criteria (Fairweather, 1967; Fairweather *et al.*, 1969), it was assumed that an unambiguous generalization from the results of this investigation would be possible.

TABLE 4.1A *Demographic Characteristics of Patient Groups: Male Patients*

Group no.[a]	Mean age	Mean years of hospitalization	Mean category of education[b]	Number married	Number paranoid
		Experimental Groups			
		Building I			
1	47.12	12.28	2.75	2	5
2	46.00	12.18	2.75	2	4
3	48.50	13.41	2.50	2	4
4	46.12	12.14	3.12	2	5
5	47.12	12.85	2.50	1	4
6	47.37	12.11	2.37	3	4
7	46.63	13.18	2.87	3	5
8	47.25	12.18	2.50	2	5
		Building II			
9	47.37	15.90	2.12	1	5
10	49.25	16.22	2.75	1	4
11	47.50	15.51	2.22	1	5
12	46.37	14.95	2.50	2	5
13	47.12	16.85	3.12	2	5
14	46.87	15.11	2.25	1	5
15	47.12	15.55	3.12	1	5
16	47.87	16.02	2.50	2	5
E Total mean	47.22	14.15	2.62	1.75	4.69
		Control Groups			
		Building I			
1	47.37	12.11	3.12	1	5
2	47.37	12.05	2.87	2	4
		Building II			
3	47.61	15.93	2.25	1	5
4	47.87	16.09	2.50	2	5
C Total mean	47.55	14.05	2.69	1.50	4.75

[a] Two group leaders (one male, one female) dropped out very early in the program and their patients were reassigned so as to maintain matching.
[b] 1: None; 2: 1–8 years; 3: 9–11 years; 4: High school grad.; 5: High school plus.

Following matching and assignment of patients to treatment conditions, student leaders were assigned to individual subgroups. Within both the 16 male and 16 female patient groups, eight male and eight female students were randomly assigned as leaders. This resulted in an experimental design with four treatment conditions: male students with male patients, male students with

TABLE 4.1B. *Demographic Characteristics of Patient Groups: Female Patients*

Group no.	Mean age	Mean years of hospitalization	Mean category of education	Number married	Number paranoid
		Experimental Groups			
		Building III			
1	46.85	12.22	2.85	2	4
2	46.28	12.54	2.00	3	4
3	47.37	12.43	3.00	4	5
4	46.88	12.32	2.75	1	5
5	46.62	12.17	2.50	3	4
6	47.00	12.01	3.00	4	5
7	46.85	12.25	3.29	4	4
8	46.62	12.19	2.00	4	5
9	46.87	12.27	2.83	2	5
10	47.28	12.70	2.42	4	4
11	36.71	12.17	2.25	4	4
12	46.62	12.20	2.00	3	4
13	36.00	12.32	2.28	2	4
14	47.25	12.31	3.12	3	4
15	46.37	12.16	3.00	4	4
16	47.25	12.79	2.71	1	4
E Total mean	46.86	12.32	2.63	3.00	4.31
		Control Groups			
		Building III			
1	46.62	12.16	2.62	4	4
2	46.00	12.01	2.22	4	4
3	46.50	12.33	2.37	4	5
4	46.22	12.17	3.37	3	4
C Total mean	46.34	12.17	2.65	3.75	4.25

female patients, female students with male patients, and female students with female patients, as well as two patient-control groups, one of each sex. Table 3.1 (p. 59) illustrates this design and indicates the number of patients and volunteers in each cell. The total number of patients was 320 with 256 Es, 128 of each sex, and 64 Cs, 32 of each sex.

Early in the program, two student leaders, one male and one female, who had been assigned to male patients, decided for personal reasons to discontinue participation. Their patients were reassigned to other groups in which attrition had occurred. Demographic matching of patients was maintained. Thus, a final total of 30 student-led patient groups participated in the experimental treatment condition. We shall now turn our attention to patient evaluation.

B. Outcome Measures

Previous research (Parloff, Kelman, & Frank, 1954; Zax & Klein, 1960) suggests that single estimates of change following treatment conditions are generally inadequate for evaluation of psychological improvement. Hence, the present study used multiple indicators of performance and behavior representing dimensions on which schizophrenics have been shown to function more poorly than normals (Buss & Lang, 1965; Lang & Buss, 1965). Such dimensions include psychophysical indices (Yates, 1961), perceptual and perceptual motor functions (Granger, 1961), measures of verbal ability (Eysenck, 1952), indicators of thought processes (Chapman, Chapman, & Miller, 1964; Maher, 1966; Payne, Ancivich, & Laverty, 1963; Weiner, 1966; Venables, 1964), and assessments of overt behavior. Measures representing each of these dimensions were administered on a pre–post basis, on the assumption that improvement would demonstrate program effectiveness.

Three considerations governed selection of outcome measures. First, the tests had to be ones to which the patients could respond. Second, only tests on which schizophrenics traditionally performed more poorly than normals were used. Finally, the full battery was compiled to reflect a broad spectrum of functions: psychomotor behavior, hypothesized to measure "speed and accuracy of central functions" (Yates, 1961); perceptual and perceptual-motor reactivity, assumed to relate to more complex cognitive variables (Granger, 1961); verbal fluency, often found to be markedly deficient in schizophrenics (Eysenck, 1952); thought processes; and actual observed behavior both on the ward and in the group sessions. The final selected measures can be grouped into two major classes: performance measures, and behavior ratings.

1. PERFORMANCE MEASURES

a. Tests of Psychomotor Retardation

1. Reaction Time 1 (RT 1)—speed of writing one's own full name (Babcock & Levy, 1940; Payne & Caird, 1967).
2. Reaction Time 2 (RT 2)—speed of copying the words "The United States of America" from a printed card (Babcock & Levy, 1940; Payne & Caird, 1967).
3. Tapping Speed (TAPS)—number of times a patient is able to tap a telegraph key in a 10-second period. The subject is presented with a telegraph key mounted on a small box and connected to an automatic counter. The key is turned on for 10 seconds, during which time *S* is instructed to tap as many times and as rapidly as he can.

b. Perceptual and Perceptual-Motor Tests

1. WAIS Digit Symbol Test (DS) (Wechsler, 1955).
2. The Stroop Color Naming Test (Stroop) (Thurstone & Mellinger, 1953). This test consists of a series of three cards, each with 100 items. Card A includes color patches which the *S* is asked to name. Card B requires that *S* read names of colors printed in black on a white background. Card C consists of names of colors, each printed in a color other than the one that its letters spell. The subject is required to name the actual color of the ink rather than to read the noncorresponding color-word. The score for each card, following Jensen (1965, 1966), is the time required to complete the naming task.

c. Verbal Fluency (VF)

Number of animals *S* can name in 1 minute.

d. Thought Processes

The Figure–Ground Confusion Test (FG) measures the ability to perceive hidden figures, theoretically related to complex thought processes (Weckowicz, 1960). This test was developed by Steer (Steer & Allen, 1960) and adapted for use with chronic schizophrenics (Weckowicz, 1960, Weckowicz & Blewett, 1959). A modified version was used in this study. The procedure consists of presenting two 16-card sets to the subject. The first set depicts common objects obscured by lines that cause figure–ground confusion (see Figure 4.1). The subject receives one point for correctly identifying a given object. The second set of cards includes pictures of the same objects, but without the lines, to identify errors due to factors other than figure–ground confusion (e.g., inattention, lack of motivation). Errors are scored only when *S* correctly names an object in set two, but not in set one.

All tests, pre- and postexperimental, were individually administered by several first-year clinical psychology graduate students and senior psychology undergraduates. The testers were trained in a single 2-hour session and practiced on each other until they mastered the administration procedures. Pretesting took place within 1 month of the start of the program. Posttesting was completed 5½ months later, during the final 2 weeks of the program. Testers at both pre- and postpoints had no knowledge of whether patients were in the E or C group.

2. BEHAVIOR RATINGS

a. Ward Behavior

The Ellsworth MACC Behavioral Adjustment Scale, Form II (Ellsworth, 1962) was completed for all patients by ward attendants in close contact with

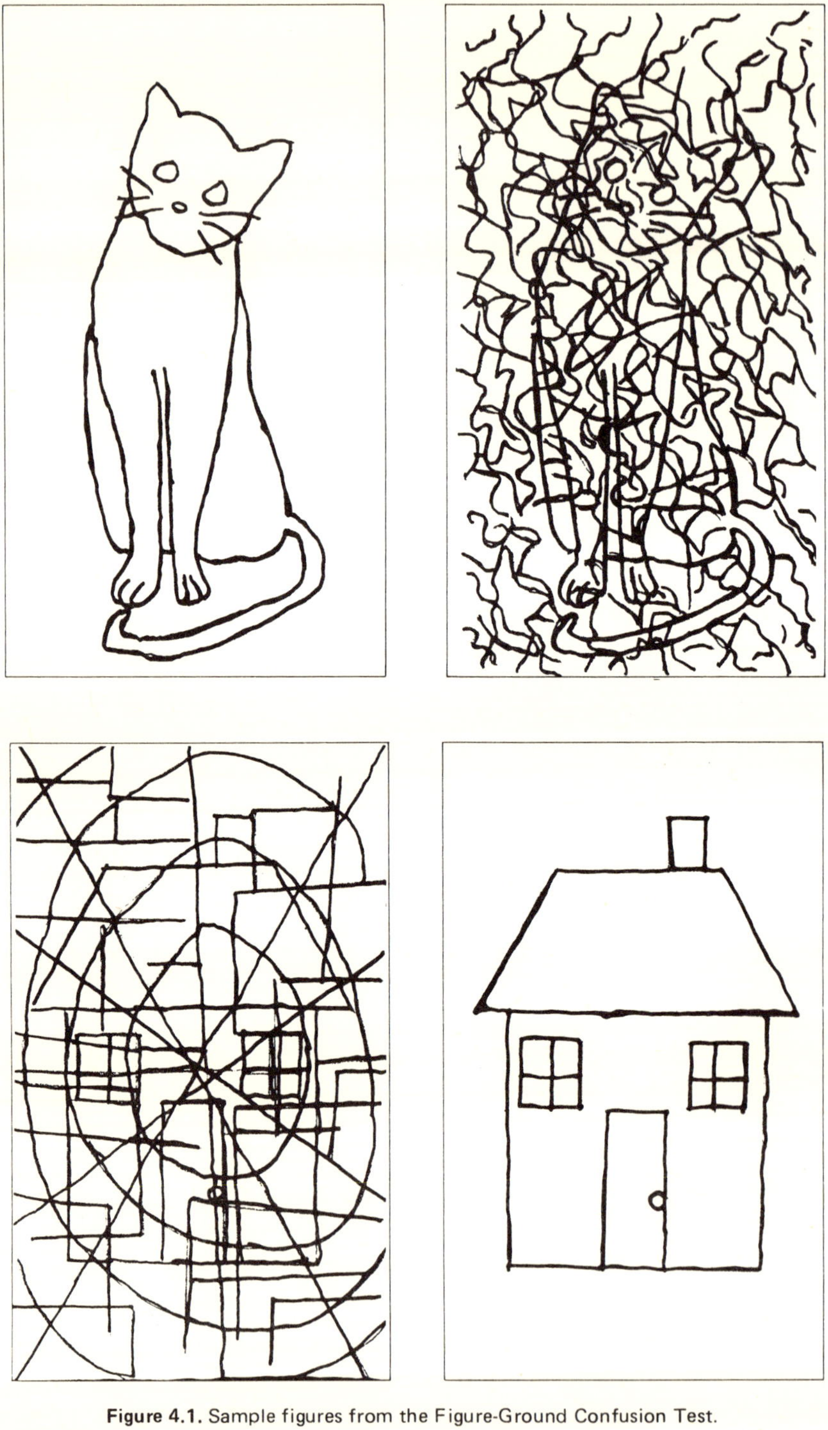

Figure 4.1. Sample figures from the Figure-Ground Confusion Test.

them. This measure consists of four factorial scales: mood, cooperation, communication, and social contact, each with four items. Raters assessed recent functioning (past 2 weeks) on each of these 16 items, using five-point scales. A total adjustment score for this measure sums all 16 ratings and, as Lyerly and Abbott (1966) state: "describes the patients' overall level of adaptability to the demands of the hospital community [p. 21]." Each patient was also rated by ward personnel on a single overall five-point evaluation of behavior ranging from "rarely good" to "almost always good" (see Table 4.2). Ward behavior ratings were made during the same time-periods, both pre- and postexperimental, during which patients were individually tested.

b. Group Behavior

The Ellsworth scale described previously was adapted for use by the student leaders to rate patients' behavior during the actual group sessions. Items were slightly reworded so as to refer to the group, rather than to the ward situation. Student leaders also completed the single overall five-point adjustment rating. The group behavior "pretest" rating was made after volunteers had met with their groups for 5 weeks, and was repeated during the last week of the program.

C. Patient Perceptions of the College-Student Volunteers

An attempt was also made to examine the chronic patients' expectations and perceptions about the college students. How are students initially seen in relation to the professional staff? Furthermore, how do these perceptions change as a result of long term contact with students? Several authors (Apfelbaum, 1958; Berzins, Geller, Rogers, & Rickers-Ovsiankina, 1966; Goldstein, 1966) have commented specifically on the importance of the patients' perception of the helping person as a factor in therapeutic change.

In order to evaluate patients' perceptions of the college students, a measure simple enough for chronic schizophrenics to follow was developed during the pilot study and administered during pre- and posttesting. This

TABLE 4.2 *Form for Single Overall Rating of Patient's Behavior on the Ward*

According to *your own* best judgment about what makes a "good" patient, this patient's overall behavior on the ward during the *past two weeks* has been:

1	2	3	4	5
Rarely good	Occasionally good	Fairly often good	Usually good	Almost always good

measure, the Patient Expectations and Perceptions Scale (PEP), includes 25 statements such as: "He advises you"; "He is critical"; "He senses your feelings" (see Table 4.3). These were read aloud to the *S* in a structured interview fashion. The interviewer first read the item and then asked if it best described a doctor or a college student, alternating the order of presentation of the response options.

Eighteen of the items were slight modifications of those listed by Apfelbaum 1958) as most characteristic of patient descriptions of therapists. Six of these fall on each of three clusters–the therapist perceived as nurturant, as a model, or as a critic (see Table 4.3). In addition, seven items were added in order

TABLE 4.3 *Pretest Distribution of Patient Endorsements for 25 PEP Items: All Patients*

	Item[a]	Frequency of doctor endorsement[b]	Frequency of college student endorsement	χ^2
1.	He advises you (N)	226	41	130.26***
2.	He is well adjusted (M)	175	93	25.01***
3.	He is critical (C)	130	138	.24
4.	He senses your feelings (N)	234	34	149.25***
5.	He is calm (M)	217	51	102.82***
6.	He is blunt (C)	128	140	.51
7.	He encourages you (N)	218	50	105.31***
8.	He gets along well with others	148	120	2.93
9.	He is clear headed (C)	191	77	34.02***
10.	He is easy to get to know (N)	130	137	.18
11.	He works hard (M)	179	89	30.22***
12.	He is hard to please (C)	115	153	5.39*
13.	He is sympathetic (N)	217	51	102.82***
14.	He is friendly (M)	158	109	8.60**
15.	He is bossy (C)	124	143	1.49
16.	He is gentle (N)	215	52	100.36***
17.	He is considerate (M)	209	58	86.21***
18.	He is self-confident (C)	175	92	25.80***
19.	He is a lot like you (SD)	91	176	27.06***
20.	He is interested in you (SD)	217	50	104.45***
21.	He is eager to help you (SD)	217	49	106.11***
22.	He likes you (SD)	171	96	21.06***
23.	He is fun to be with (SD)	82	185	39.73***
24.	You like him (SD)	165	102	14.87***
25.	You would like to be like him (SD)	148	120	2.93

[a] N: Nurturant cluster; M: Model cluster; C: Critic cluster; SD: New social distance items.

[b] Total frequency may vary from item to item since some patients could not always make a forced choice for some items.

*$p < .05$. **$p < .01$. ***$p < .001$.

to test the hypothesis that patients perceive nonprofessionals as closer to themselves in the "social hierarchy." An example of the new social distance items, which appear as numbers 19–25 in Table 4.3, is: "He is fun to be with."

While the main reason for using the PEP was to determine how patients' attitudes toward students changed following contact with them in the program, the measure also provided an opportunity to identify patients' initial stereotypic views of college students before the experiment started. Such information is potentially useful in determining whether the effectiveness of a program involving a new type of helping agent, is due in part to an initially favorable view of the helpers. In that vein, the analysis of the total group able to complete the preexperimental PEP responses ($N = 268$) is presented here to portray the patients' initial image of college students. So far as is known, few, or none of the patients had any prior contact with student volunteers. Accordingly, their "preexperimental" responses, comparing students to physicians, should reflect stereotypic views of the former.

Had chance alone guided patient responses for each of the 25 PEP items, students and physicians would have been selected for 50% of the time. Departure of the actual selection pattern from theoretical expectancy was tested for significance, for each individual item. The results of this analysis are presented in Table 4.3 The actual endorsements did *not* follow a chance pattern; significant differences in choice were found for 19 of the 25 items. On almost all of these, the doctor was preferred to the student. In comparison with students, doctors were perceived by the patients to be significantly more: giving of advice, well adjusted, hard-working, sympathetic, friendly, gentle, considerate, self-confident, interested in the patient, eager to help, liking of the patient, and liked. Students were seen as more difficult to please. Students were significantly preferred to physicians on only two items. These were: "fun to be with" and "like me." These findings suggest that students were either not readily identifiable entities to patients, preexperimently, or, if so, they were not favorably regarded.

Knowing the preprogram attitudes of the patients to helpers allows us to assess the extent to which initial positive attitudes influenced program effects. In this case, initial patient attitudes toward students were unfavorable; hence, observed positive program effects cannot be attributed to that source. However, the patients did perceive students as relatively closer than doctors in social status, a factor which Guerney (1969) has observed may strengthen the students' position as a "significant other" or potential social reinforcer. In that sense, the patients were indeed able to perceive students in a "like me" manner, beforehand.

Change in patient attitudes to students as a function of their participation in the program is considered with the other patient data in Chapter 5.

II. MEETINGS AND PROCESS EVALUATION

A. Patient Meetings and Process Measures

Regularized group meetings involving a single student leader and eight patients were at the heart of the program. Each student initially met with his group for 1 hour, one evening a week, beginning in late November or early December and continuing until early February. From early February until the end of the academic year (the second week in May), meetings were held twice weekly. The program was capped by a massive outdoor picnic in late May involving all student leaders, patients, and hospital staff. The total number of meetings for any given group varied from 26 to 33 1-hour sessions over the 5½-month program period. This variation was due to vicissitudes in the group leaders' schedules, as, for example, vacations, examination periods, or illness. Students were quite faithful in keeping to their meeting schedules with patients.

Student leaders were not, at the outset, told specifically what to do in these meetings. Their principal instruction was to do whatever they could to foster verbal and nonverbal communication and interaction among patients and between patients and those with whom they had contact. What students actually did in the groups was determined by factors such as their own interests and styles, the interests and functioning level of group members, and pragmatism. Where a student had special interests and skills in dramatics, photography, music, or crafts, that interest typically found its way into the groups' activity. While there was little initial instruction about what specifically to do with patients, practical questions of handling, management, and motivation of patients were frequently considered during the group supervisory sessions. Often, in such meetings, students who were particularly successful with an approach described their experiences for their peers. Where indicated, specific suggestions were made by the program consultants to students running into difficulties with their groups.

Conditions of the student–patient meetings, in terms of what rooms were available, their location, patient transportation problems, and available materials and supplies were far from ideal. These matters are reserved for fuller discussion in Chapter 7, where the "human" side of the study is considered.

Students kept reasonably detailed records of the activities of their patient group through a specially devised group process schedule called the Group Activities Form (GAF). This schedule (see Table 4.4) consisted of nine categories, each defined for the student rater, spanning a broad spectrum of possible group activities: eating, talking, musical activities, listening, artistic activities, table games, physical activities, individual activities, and quiet times. The form was filled out for each third of the total experience (approximately after each 10 sessions). For each of the nine process categories, the student leader indicated the percentage of time spent by the group in that activity during the period covered by the report, whether the activity was group or leader-initiated, and how much the group enjoyed the activity. He also listed the names of the patients who participated in each rated activity. Two additional general rating scales were included at the end of the process form. One was a five-point scale evaluating how well the group as a whole had done during the time period covered, and the other, a seven-point scale, evaluated the extent to which the group had improved or gone downhill since the preceding rating period.

The process form served multiple purposes. First, it provided the basis for describing the overall nature of the group transaction, group variability in this regard, and changes over the course of the program. It also constituted a framework within which two potentially important related questions could be considered: (1) the relation between student personality and attitude variables and the actual interaction process, and (2) the relation of process to patient outcome.

B. Student Supervisory Meetings

The second type of meeting involved all 30 student leaders subdivided into four equal groups and the first two authors (J.R. and J.C.) who served as consultants and supervisors for them. Each author worked with two subgroups of 7-8 student leaders, meeting with them regularly for 1 hour a week. Occasionally, there were additional joint meetings involving both supervisors and all 30 group leaders. As earlier noted, the regular supervisory meetings were discussion-oriented rather than didactic, and covered various matters. Administrative problems such as availability of rooms, materials, supplies, and hospital policy were often considered. Concerns about patients were prominent, particularly those who did not seem to respond in the group setting. Stratagems for promoting patient participation, both those that worked and those that did not, were frequently considered. Matters of patient handling and the role of the student leader attracted much attention. At times, students' personal concerns about their own role or style were discussed.

The full cycle of these discussion sessions reveals a generally orderly progression through three identifiable stages, granting considerable individual variability. The early discussion meetings featured much student expression of anxiety about working in a mental hospital, a sense of shock and upset about the seemingly extreme deterioration of many patients, and ample verbalized hostility toward the institution, accompanied by strong negative feelings about the conditions under which chronic patients live. This was a "culture-shock" period. During this phase, and even later, there was an undercurrent of feeling

TABLE 4.4 *Group Activities Form (GAF)*

Name

Date

Number of people usually in your group sessions

We are asking you to fill out the following form in order that we can get some more specific idea of what you and your group have been doing for the past several weeks. On the next page is a list of activities which we hope include most of the activities which you have engaged in. Please notice the "other" category. Quite possibly some of your activities will not seem to you to fit adequately into any of the other categories, and if so, please describe them in the space provided. Note: you are by no means expected to have done any particular one of these things, either up to now or at any time in the future. If this list gives you some ideas, fine, but don't feel that because you haven't done something on the list that you ought to have done it.

1. We would like to have a rough estimate of the amount of time you have spent at the various things you have done. To that end, please indicate in the appropriate space beside each category the per cent of your time that has been spent at that kind of activity. *Don't refine your estimates more closely than units of 5%. Please make sure the total adds up to 100%.*

2. For each of the categories you have indicated you have spent time at, please also indicate which of you, the group, yourself, or both customarily initiates the activity.

3. Also, for each of these, indicate how well you feel *the group as a whole* enjoys the activity, on a scale from 1 to 5, as below:

1—strongly dislikes 2—mildly dislikes 3—neutral, indifferent
4—mildly enjoys 5—strongly enjoys

4. Sometimes when the group as a whole is doing something, not all patients are involved. In the last column, put the *names of the group members* usually engaged in this activity.

	Percentage of time spent at an activity	Who usually initiates (you, the group, or both?)	How much the group liked the activity (from 1, strongly dislikes to 5 strongly likes)	Who (name) usually participates in the activity?
Eating Including preparation of food.				
Talking You talk all the time, of course, but this refers to those times when, though there may be something else going on, *the most important thing is the conversation.*				
Musical activities Playing an instrument, singing—this category includes times when the patients are *actively* engaged in musical activities.				
Listening Times when the group is *passive,* listening to a record, a poem				

	Percentage of time spent at an activity	Who usually initiates (you, the group, or both?)	How much the group liked the activity (from 1, strongly dislikes to 5 strongly likes)	Who (name) usually participates in the activity?
you are reading, an instrument you are playing, etc.				
Artistic activities Painting, drawing, sculpting, any of the fine arts activities.				
Table games Patients are seated and engaged in organized *group activity*—bingo, cards, etc.				
Physical activity Times when the patients are physically active—playing darts, bowling, dancing, etc.				
Individual activities Individual patients doing things *alone*—puzzles, reading.				
Quiet times Patients are not engaged in conversation or activities.				
Other Please feel free to put down any other category or activity that you feel doesn't adequately fit into one of the categories above. Please try to explain it so that what you mean is clear.				

Total________%.

Part 2

1. According to your own best judgment about what makes a "good group," how would you rate your group's behavior during the past few weeks.

1	2	3	4	5
Rarely good	Occasionally good	Fairly often good	Usually good	Almost always good

2. Using the seven-point scale below, in which "4" equals no change, indicate how much, and in what direction, you think your group's behavior has changed since your last rating.

1	2	3	4	5	6	7
Considerably worse	Somewhat worse	Slightly worse	No change	Slightly improved	Somewhat improved	Considerably improved

among some student leaders that formal protest or social action, directed against the administration of Rochester State Hospital, should be developed.

A second phase of concern during the middle stages of the program, featured preoccupations about what, if anything, the students could hope to achieve, given the overwhelming adversity of the life circumstances of patients and the dismal hospital living conditions. The initial attitudes of optimism, enthusiasm, and a promise of "cure," had yielded to stark reality and to the onset of a pervasive pessimism. During this period, a number of students pressed for specific instruction from supervisors in methods and techniques that would quickly lead to positive patient change. Students seemed to believe that the supervisors were holding back on the "real" professionally guarded cure-techniques, and, that if they could only be instructed in these, immediate positive change would take place in patients.

In the final phase of the program, discussion centered around a realistic assessment of accomplishment and failures. Students were better able to perceive positive change, albeit in limited rather than earth-shaking ways as originally hoped. During this final period, problems of termination, separation from patients, and concerns about their future, were very much in the forefront.

III. STUDENTS

A. The Volunteer Sample and Control Groups

1. VOLUNTEER SAMPLE

This section of the chapter describes the student-leader sample and presents data about student motivations for participating in the practicum program. The initial decision to contact psychology majors, in announcing the new practicum course sequence and inviting applicants, was dictated more by their prospectively high interest and the fact that they were quickly and easily located, than by the specifics of their prior training. In fact, we believed that the group could, in principle, have included other than psychology majors. For example, Poser's (1966) student leaders had no previous psychology background whatever. Two factors weighed on our decision to use only juniors and seniors: First, students do not become identified as departmental majors until late in the sophomore year; and second, in a limited-enrollment course, likely to be oversubscribed, advanced students are normally given priority in registration.

Within the first several weeks of the semester, students were given a questionnaire asking them to indicate why they had enrolled in the program. Frankness and honesty of response were encouraged; this was perhaps easier because students had already been admitted to the program. By far, the most frequent reason cited was to help in determining a vocational choice. A fair number of students had been contemplating future work in the mental health fields and believed that the program would provide an opportunity for first-hand experience to clarify their thinking. Specific career alternatives under consideration were varied. Some students were trying to decide between psychology and related professions. Others, already committed to attending graduate school in psychology, were uncertain as to whether to specialize in clinical or experimental psychology. Some who planned to go on to medical school thought the experience would be helpful in deciding whether or not to specialize in psychiatry.

Another strong attraction to the program was its service aspects. The students wanted to do something "relevant" and practical to help others. They took these service obligations with deadly seriousness. A number of students were "activists" who wished to channel social protest into a constructive form. Several were attracted by the particular combination of the challenges that the course seemed to offer. The screening interview and early discussions had emphasized the heavy amount of work involved both in academic and practicum aspects of the course. Some students noted that the opportunity to evaluate their aptitudes in both of these areas was attractive. Another reason given for interest in the program was the chance to become involved in a smaller, more personalized learning situation. Similarly, students were eager to engage in a practical application of what they had "acquired" in prior psychology courses; they wanted to avoid simple "book learning." Finally, several students wanted to fill major-area requirements in psychology, though none reported this as a primary reason for taking the course. From the initial description of the tasks required, the students were all fully aware that there were easier ways to accomplish the latter goal.

2. CONTROLS

There were two groups of student controls. One (SC I) consisted of 30 junior and senior psychology majors demographically similar to the experimental student-leader group. These students had indicated on the questionnaire sent out the preceding summer (see Figure 2.1, p. 52) that they would have liked taking the course, but were unable to do so, due either to prior course commitments or to schedule conflicts. Neither of these responses was surprising, since the solicitation letter was sent out late in the summer, after many students had already preregistered for fall courses.

This control group was selected because of its close similarity to the student-leader group in interest in the mental health field, age, and prior training and course background in psychology. It was, perhaps, the most similar group to the volunteers available on campus. Its primary purpose was as a control in assessing changes in attitudes and self-perceptions as a function of the practicum experience. Essentially, the question asked was, "Other things the same, what effect do the course and practicum experiences have on one's self-perception and attitudes toward mental health and related concepts?"

A second student control group (SC II) consisted of 61 sophomores, juniors, and seniors drawn from a large introductory psychology lecture course. The group included 26 females (22 sophomores and 4 juniors) and 35 males (1 senior, 7 juniors, and 27 sophomores); thus, 49 of 61 SC II's were sophomores. The mean age of the group was 18.93 years and the age range 18–21. Thus, SC II was both more diverse and less senior than the student-leader group. It was chosen as a sample of the undergraduate population at large. Its primary purpose was to provide a base of comparison for the student E-group on the attitude and personality measures used to evaluate them. The issue at stake was whether program volunteers differed from "typical college students" on those dimensions. SC II represented the latter, since more than 90% of undergraduates at the University of Rochester take the Introductory Psychology course.

B. Student Evaluation Measures

Student Es and Cs were evaluated on a broad spectrum of "therapeutic talent," personality, and attitude measures yielding a total of 85 test and subtest scores. Depending on the questions asked, either SC I or SC II was the appropriate control group. In the next section, the student evaluation measures are reported and, where necessary, their nature and the conditions of their administration are more fully described. The time sequence for the administration of these assessment procedures is also indicated. One point that bears emphasis is that students were advised from the very start that extensive research evaluation, including evaluation of themselves, was to be an ongoing and major aspect of the program. This point was stated in the initial soliciting letter (see Figure 2.1), repeated at the time of the screening interviews, and brought up frequently during the earlier didactic phases of the course.

1. THERAPEUTIC TALENT MEASURES

The characteristics of "nonpossessive" warmth, "genuineness" or self-congruence, and accurate empathy, have been found by Truax and Carkhuff to be related to therapeutic effectiveness (Chapter I). Truax's early findings (1961) suggested that these three variables discussed on page 29 were significant interpersonal dimensions that related positively to successful patient outcomes. Although the authors have subsequently questioned the meaning of several of these ratings (Chinsky & Rappaport, 1970; Rappaport & Chinsky, 1971), at the time, it was predicted that volunteer warmth, empathy, and genuineness would correlate positively with patient improvement.

In order to obtain these measures, the following procedure was invoked: Between Sessions 15 and 20, a point at which the group sessions have stabilized, according to Truax and Carkhuff, each volunteer tape-recorded one patient group meeting. A 4-minute segment was randomly selected from the second half of each tape, Each segment was rated on the Truax dimensions of accurate empathy, nonpossessive warmth, and congruence by separate pairs of female judges. Each rater team made only one set of ratings for each set of tape segments in order to assure independence of ratings (Chinsky & Rappaport, 1970). Thus, there were three separate sets of rater pairs, one for each of the three variables.

Each rater pair was first given a copy of the relevant scale to study and then assigned to rate practice materials. Raters were told to do their ratings in accord with the scale descriptions, but were not instructed on what ratings to give any specific segment. Training continued until the raters agreed within one scale-point on at least 75% of their ratings. The average practice time needed to meet this criterion was about 8 hours. Ratings on the experimental materials were done individually, approximately 1 week after training ended. Since the data for these three sets of judgments came from a taped segment of an actual group session, no comparable control measure was available.

A second therapeutic talent measure, also described in Chapter 1, is the Whitehorn and Betz (1954) A–B scale, essentially a measure of interaction style. Prior data cited suggested that A therapists were more effective than B therapists with schizophrenic patients. Such data justified extension of the test of this relation to the college student volunteers in the present study. Two issues were at stake here: (1) whether the selected volunteer sample differed in A–B scores from typical college students as represented in SC II, and (2) whether A-scores were positively correlated with indices of patient improvement. A constraint attached to this set of analyses is that the A–B scale was standardized on males; the present student sample included both males and females.

The A–B scale was given, in group administration, to the student volunteers and SC II well before the program started. It was given together with other tests during one of a series of group testing sessions. A schematic time table summarizing the student testing procedures is presented in Figure 4.2.

Another approach to the study of the effective college student volunteer stems from the work of Goodman (1965, 1969) who developed a structured behavioral technique to assess understanding, openness, and accepting-warmth. This procedure, known as the Group Assessment of Interpersonal Traits (GAIT) has been discussed in detail on page 31. Volunteers participated in a GAIT session in like-sexed groups of eight, shortly before the patient program began.

	Pre-practicum		*Practicum*				*Post-practicum*
	Sept.	Dec.				May	
	Session Number: 1	4	10	15	20	30	
SE *N* = 30	SD and ACL (1) Pencil and paper personality measures GAIT	SD ACL (2)	GAF (1)	Truax tapes	GAF (2)	GAF (3)	SD ACL (3)
SC I *N* = 30	SD and ACL (1)	SD ACL (2)					SD ACL (3)
SC II *N* = 61	SD and ACL (1) Pencil and paper personality measures	SD ACL (2)					SD ACL (3)

Figure 4.2 Time sequence for testing student-leader and control groups.

There was no control group for this measure; it was used exclusively within the E-group to predict patient success.

2. PERSONALITY AND ATTITUDE COMPARISONS

Direct comparisons of students who participated in the program and their controls were carried out for two classes of measures—personality and attitude indices. Among the former was a cluster of standardized tests including the following: Jackson's Personality Research Form (PRF) (Jackson, 1965) providing measures of 20 personality-related variables each reflecting a need category within Murray's system (1935) for analyzing thematic responses; a measure of locus of control based on the Internal-External locus of Control Scale (Rotter, 1966); Chapin's Social Insight Test (1942); Jourard's Self-Disclosure Inventory (1964), each of the latter purportedly measuring the variable named in its title; and Wrightsmann's Philosophies of Human Nature Scale (1964).

To assess initial attitudes and attitude change over the program period, two additional measures were used both with Es and Cs: an adjective checklist (ACL) based on a format developed by Gough and Heilbrun (1965) and a semantic differential attitude scale (Osgood, Suci, & Tannenbaum, 1957), containing a broad spectrum of concepts related to mental illness and to the mental hospital patient, specially adapted for the present study.

The ACL was administered with two different sets of instructions. Respondents were first asked to check adjectives to describe themselves, and then to check adjectives describing the "typical mental hospital patient." Twenty-two of the 24 ACL scales (excluding "total number of adjectives" and "counseling readiness") were used to score self-attitudes. Only the "favorable" and the "unfavorable" scales were used to score attitudes toward mental hospital patients.

The semantic differential (SD) included nine concepts, each rated on 14 scales. The concepts were: myself, mental patients, mental hospital, volunteer groups, psychologists, nurses, average person, mental illness, and psychotherapy. The 14 scales were:

effective–ineffective
good–bad
healthy–sick
relaxed–tense
friendly–unfriendly
interesting–boring
pleasant–unpleasant
understandable–mysterious
helpful–harmful
warm–cold
safe–dangerous
strong–weak
active–passive
predictable–unpredictable

The favorable adjective on each scale, as determined by at least 80% agreement of five independent raters, is listed first. Placing the favorable pole on the left or right was randomized in actual administration. Concept scores were obtained by summing scale ratings in the favorable direction.

Thus, of the full student-test battery described in this chapter, different measures, serving different purposes, were taken by different subgroups. Two, the GAIT and the Truax-Carkhuff, were taken only by Es and were used exclusively as predictors of student effectiveness with patients. Three others, the ACL, the semantic-differential and the A-B were used both as predictors and for initial comparison of the characteristics of student leaders versus SC II. Five other tests—the PRF, locus of control, self-discolosure, philosophy of human nature, and social insight tests—were used only for initial group comparisons. Finally, two measures, the semantic differential and the ACL were used to compare student leaders to the similar SC I. This second control group was used to establish a baseline for evaluating change in student attitudes as a function of program participation.

The schedule for testing student *S*s was as follows: The semantic differential and the ACL were given to the student E-group and both C-groups three times each: at the very beginning of the course, 1 month after contact with patients began, and at the end of the practicum experience. All other personality tests were given to Es and SC IIs during three separate group administrations between the third and seventh week of the course, before practicum work started. The GAIT session for Es only, was held after all other group testing had been completed and immediately before practicum activities started. The Truax-Carkhuff ratings for Es only were based on taped excerpts from a single group meeting after not less than 15 or more than 20 group sessions. Figure 4.2 is a "flow chart" depicting the student-testing sequence along a time axis.

A further, albeit secondary, empirical, interest in the student test data was to examine interrelations among personality and attitude variables included in the battery.

Chapter 5

RESEARCH EVALUATION: PATIENTS

The research findings of the study are reported in two chapters, this one for patient data and Chapter 6 for student data. Patient results are presented in several sections. First, attendance at group meetings is reported and experimental *S*s are designated "attenders" (EAs) or "nonattenders" (ENAs). Total E and C groups, EAs, and ENAs, are next compared on pretest measures, followed by the central patient-change analyses. Program effectiveness evaluations are divided into two major sections: within group changes for both E and C groups, and differential change between groups. Separate comparisons of several subgroups are also presented. The next major section presents data on relations between demographic and pretest characteristics and patient improvement scores. A final section deals with changes in patient views of college students.

I. ATTENDANCE AND PROCESS DATA

A. Attendance

The project's stance toward patient attendance at the group meetings is fairly described by the term "semi-optional." Typically, patients were approached by ward attendants prior to each scheduled meeting, reminded of the meeting, and invited to attend. Patients were never forced to attend! This orientation and the calculated effort to respect the patient's right to self-determination created some unexpected complications for evaluation of the data. In effect, our stance toward patient attendance permitted the attitudes of ward attendants to become an important factor in determining whether or not patients came to meetings. Although data on attendants' attitudes were not collected, our distinct impression was that patient attendance on a given day was, at least partially, a function of which ward attendant happened to be on duty. Attendants with favorable attitudes to the program generated high attendance rates; those with negative attitudes made for nonattendance. This point will be developed more fully in a subsequent section (see Chapter 7) dealing with program impact on the hospital.

Since the ultimate question to be resolved before major data analyses could be undertaken, was: "How many patients attended meetings *regularly* and may therefore be considered to have participated in the program?", actual patient attendance was an important variable. The key in answering this question lies in defining the word "regularly." The extreme case of patients who attended no meetings, or only one or two, is an easy one. Such patients were *not* functionally part of the program. However, a vague "middle ground" existed. Should patients who attended one-third, one-half, or three-quarters of the meetings be classified as bona fide attenders?

An arbitrary decision was made to classify patients as "attenders" if they were at two-thirds or more of their scheduled group meetings. There were two justifications for this "cut-point." First, it represented a substantial bloc of meetings and thus, significant exposure to the program. Second, there was a natural falling off in the attendance curve such that only 11 patients (5%) fell into the next lowest attendance category, 50–65%. A total of 161 patients (63%) attended two-thirds or more of their scheduled group meetings. Of these, 138 (54% of the total patient sample) actually attended 90% or more of the meetings. This group of 161 is hereafter called the "experimental attenders" (EAs). The major outcome analyses to follow are based primarily on this group. Of the remaining 95 (37%) of the E group who were nonattenders (ENAs), and therefore excluded from the major substantive analyses, 67 (71% of the ENAs) attended fewer than a third of the sessions. Table 5.1 presents patient attendance data for the total E group, based on the ratio of meetings actually attended to total number of meetings.

Within the total E group of 256, it was possible to retest 222 (87%) at the end of the program. If a patient could not be tested the first time, a second attempt was always made. Thus, 34 patients (13%) failed twice to complete posttesting. Of this group, four were out of the hospital on family-care, five were too ill physically to be tested, seven were too upset psychologically, five had eloped from the hospital, and 13 refused testing. Of particular interest, no EAs and only one C patient missed the posttesting. In other words, 33 of the 34 posttest failures came from the ENA group of 95 *S*s. This finding takes on greater significance because the testers were unaware of the groups to which

TABLE 5.1 *Patient Attendance Record: E Group*

Percentage of total meetings attended	*N*
32% or less	67
33-49%	17
50-65%	11
66-89%	23
90% or more	138
Total *N*	256

patients were assigned. Indeed, the entities EA and ENA did not even exist at the posttest point.

B. Process

Student leaders completed the group activities form (GAF) (see Chapter 4, Table 4.4), three times during the course of the program. This form recorded the amount of time spent by each group in various activities potentially available to them and served as an index of group interaction process.

Two classes of activities, talking and conversation, with an overall frequency of 27.30%, and table games, at 23.83%, occupied more than half of the groups' time. Two other categories, eating and food preparation (12.44%) and artistic activites (11.66%), were of intermediate frequency. The remaining categories were of considerably lower frequency ranging from 1.20% (musical activity) to 6.93% (passive listening). Subperiod and overall mean percentage of time spent by groups in various activities are summarized In Table 5.2

The process data, as presented, are averaged for all 30 groups. As can be seen from the category-dispersion estimates in Table 5.2, there was substantial variability among groups in several process categories, particularly talking, table games, and artistic activity. Of the relatively high-frequency activities, the one that was most stable and predictable was eating and food preparation. For chronic hospitalized patients, such activity is salient, important, and serves as a good point of entrée and communication for the outsider. Many students, especially in the early stages of the program, found that foodmaking activities and food consumption was a good bet to draw patients out and to enable them to interact.

II. PRETEST DATA

Both because of sharp time constraints and the substantial number of patients, about 400, who had to be individually tested within several weeks, it

TABLE 5.2 *Mean Percentage of Time Spent at Group Activities for Each Third and Total Program*

Activity	Mean percentage				
	First GAF	Second GAF	Final GAF	Total mean	Standard deviation
Food preparation and eating	12.7	10.6	13.3	12.4	4.6
Talking	26.0	28.5	27.3	27.3	20.3
Musical activities	1.0	1.0	1.2	1.2	1.9
Listening	8.5	5.8	6.1	6.8	7.3
Artistic activities	11.3	14.0	9.9	11.6	15.7
Table games	21.5	24.6	25.1	23.8	17.6
Physical activities	4.6	5.0	8.1	5.9	7.6
Individual activities	2.6	3.2	2.5	2.7	4.1
Quiet times	4.5	4.1	3.9	4.1	5.6
Other	7.3	3.0	2.2	4.1	

was not possible to match E and C groups beforehand on the basis of the 16 performance and behavioral pretest scores. Following Fairweather (1967, 1969) it was assumed that close matching of E and C on the five basic demographic variables described on page 65, would yield roughly comparable scores for E and C on the criterion pretest measures. This assumption was examined statistically by t ratios, testing the significance of the differences between E and C group means on all 16 pretest measures. The analyses presented in Table 5.3 demonstrate that the assumption is not, in fact, tenable. Significant differences, each favoring (indicating *better* initial status) Cs, were found on 6 of the 16 comparisons. Moreover, Cs were *directionally* superior on 15 of the 16 measures. Clearly demographic comparability of groups did not, in this case, assure comparable pretest status. Table 5.3 also presents a structurally comparable set of analyses of pretest data, substituting EAs for the full E-group. This substitution only made an already severe problem worse. In the new analysis, nine significant differences and 15 of the 16 *directional* differences, favored Cs. Thus, EAs were even more poorly matched to Cs than was the total E-group. This point is further documented by direct comparisons of EAs and ENAs on the criterion pretest measures (Rappaport, 1968), in that ENAsshad significantly better scores on nine of the 16 measures.

As an alternative to variable by variable comparisons of the initial status of the several E-groups versus Cs, global examination of such differences was carried out using discriminant function analysis. In essence, this technique weighs and recombines separate component pretest scores to yield a composite, and then compares the two groups in question on the composite. Using this technique, EAs were once again found to have a significantly poorer overall initial status than Cs, the probability being less than 3 in 1000 that these were chance differences.

The failure to have achieved a satisfactory pretest matching of Es and Cs was both perplexing and embarrassing. It was damaging to the basic design of the study and necessitated a series of improvisations, none initially anticipated, and

TABLE 5.3 *Pretest Comparisons of All Experimentals and Experimental Attenders with Controls*

Measure	All Es versus Cs *t*	All Es[a] Mean	All Es[a] *SD*	Cs[b] Mean	Cs[b] *SD*	EAs[c] Mean	EAs[c] *SD*	EAs versus Cs *t*
RT 1[d]	1.99*	14.54	15.36	10.57	6.98	15.97	18.08	2.29*
RT 2[d]	1.52	29.36	25.40	24.15	16.73	32.65	26.50	2.31*
TAPS	−2.48*	37.37	17.12	43.44	17.65	36.90	18.38	−2.43*
DS	−2.54*	19.30	13.71	24.36	14.99	17.52	13.86	−3.23**
VF	−1.57	10.76	5.39	11.94	4.83	10.12	5.56	−2.26*
Stroop A[d]	.63	86.02	69.96	79.61	70.17	90.87	81.39	.94
Stroop B[d]	.17	121.26	65.86	119.32	117.50	122.76	57.34	.28
Stroop C[d]	2.56*	233.11	121.31	189.98	79.24	235.39	123.70	2.57*
Stroop total[d]	2.70**	430.33	189.47	358.95	124.99	437.01	200.14	2.73**
Figure ground confusion	−.22	7.89	3.14	7.98	2.86	7.52	3.24	−.99
MACC mood	−.35	15.56	2.99	15.72	3.12	15.51	3.11	−.44
MACC cooperation	−1.09	14.24	3.82	14.83	3.48	13.84	3.79	−1.75
MACC commun.	−2.10*	13.60	4.08	14.81	3.51	12.82	4.17	−3.27**
MACC social contact	− .22	12.31	4.32	12.45	4.20	11.64	4.24	−1.25
MACC total adjustment	−1.05	55.66	12.76	57.58	11.78	53.79	12.90	−1.97*
Single overall rating	.64	3.91	1.03	3.81	.99	3.91	1.04	.58

[a]*N* varies from 239 to 205. [b]*N* varies from 63 to 53.
[c]*N* varies from 161 to 141. [d]Lower Scores mean better performance.
$*p < .05$. $**p < .01$.

each less than fully satisfactory. Considerable thought and effort was invested in the matching procedure beforehand, and the method selected seemed defensible not only at the time, but even in retrospect. Unfortunately, the facts of the situation are otherwise. Despite considerable effort, it is difficult even after the fact, to identify sources of systematic error that could account for the pretest differences between Es and Cs. However unsatisfactory or unenlightening it may be to say so, the authors consider it likely that the pretest matching breakdown was essentially a chance phenomenon. Whatever the explanation, it is clear that this breakdown had serious, negative implications for all subsequent data analyses.

These pretest findings raise questions about the future use of demographic criteria for selection of "comparable" patient groups. Fairweather's suggestion (1967, 1969) that the variables of age, length of hospitalization, and diagnosis are a sufficient matching basis to ensure group comparability on other demographic measures, cannot be comfortably extrapolated to matching groups on independent performance measures as well.

Intensification of the original E-C prescore differences, when ENAs were excluded from the analysis is easier to understand. Initially, the ENAs were functioning better than the EAs and subsequent findings must be interpreted in that context. Within the total E-group, patients who scored more poorly on the criterion pretests (EAs) were probably more withdrawn, apathetic, and retarded in their performance and behavior.

When attendants came to take such patients to the group meetings, they were more likely to have complied unquestioningly. By contrast, the relatively more intact patient (ENA) probably was better able to perceive and to resist a somewhat unstructured and thus, to him, potentially dangerous new situation. That the situation was seen as dangerous is suggested in the fact (see page 72) that patients initially judged college students to be more critical and less nurturant than physicians. Although that finding may, in part, imply positive feelings for physicians, it also reflects patients' perception of potential threat from unknown college students. So it is understandable that the ENAs resisted attendance. This resistance among ENAs was also evident from the posttest data since 33 ENAs and no EAs missed testing.

For at least two reasons, chance, and the dropping out of relatively more intact patients, the EA and C groups were markedly mismatched on pretest criteria. This necessitated revising the strategy for program evaluation to weigh more heavily both on within-group analyses of change and the use of smaller, more closely matched subgroups from the initially selected total E and C groups to minimize problems created by the initial mismatching.

III. MAJOR OUTCOME EVALUATIONS

A. Changes within the Experimental and Control Groups

1. PERFORMANCE MEASURES

A way of evaluating program effects that assumed greater importance after systematic pretest mismatches had been identified,was to test the significance of prepost change scores separately for EAs and Cs. This was done using *t* tests for correlated means (Winer, 1962) for each of the 10 test-performance measures.

The total EA group improved significantly on eight of the 10 performance measures, while Cs improved significantly on only three. Male EAs improved significantly on seven of 10 performance tests, while male Cs improved significantly on only one and did significantly more poorly on another. For the female groups, EAs improved significantly on seven of 10 measures and Cs on four of 10. Thus, in comparison to Cs, EAs showed greater improvement, particularly so for the males. Table 5.4 presents the within-group changes in *performance* tests for Es and Cs based on the total sample, and male and female subgroups.

Summarizing, on test performance measures, EAs showed greater improvement than Cs. This differential improvement, while true for the total EA group and both sex subgroups individually, was strongest for male EAs, where significant improvement was found on seven of 10 measures in comparison to only one of 10 for Cs. The male C-group was the only subgroup in which Cs were basically stable from pre- to posttest. The significant improvement of female and total EAs was occasionally paralleled by some, though typically less significant C-improvement. The foregoing set of analyses provides the first evidence that the program was differentially effective for different subgroups. Further supporting data are presented in Section C.

Looking beyond the differential improvement of the E and C groups, to its specific nature, EAs showed significant reduction in psychomotor retardation, a classic and, ordinarily, highly change-resistant measure used to evaluate schizophrenics (Shakow, 1962). EAs also improved significantly in perceptual and perceptual-motor functions, suggesting increased responsiveness to the environment. In the male EA versus male C comparison, Cs either remained stable or performed more poorly on all posttest measures except for the Figure-Ground Confusion Test on which both groups improved. Improvement on this measure may be due to a test–retest effect rather than to a program effect. Overall, EAs especially males, demonstrated an "awakening" characterized by greater alert-

TABLE 5.4 *t Tests for Pre-Post Change in Test Performance Measures*

						Stroop				
	RT 1	RT 2	TAPS	DS	VF	A	B	C	TOTAL	FG
All EAs[a]	2.93**	2.49*	1.37	4.69**	1.75	2.11*	3.87**	3.39*	3.80**	4.98**
All controls[b]	−1.05[g]	1.36	.53	2.09*	.18	1.76	1.69	1.97	2.61*	3.55**
Male EAs[c]	2.41*	2.39*	− .35	3.48**	1.92	1.70	3.57**	2.84**	3.14**	4.00**
Male controls[d]	− .97[g]	−.54	−3.19*	− .38	− .97	1.75	1.67	1.19	1.30	2.73**
Female EAs[e]	1.89	.88	3.08**	3.14**	.22	2.07*	2.03	2.02*	2.27*	3.00**
Female controls[f]	− .45	1.26	2.42*	4.15**	1.11	1.48	1.30	1.65	2.42*	2.34*

[a] N varies from 161 to 126. [b] N varies from 63 to 53.
[c] N varies from 86 to 71. [d] N varies from 32 to 26.
[e] N varies from 75 to 55. [f] N varies from 31 to 27.
[g] Negative t indicates a decrease in performance. $*p < .05$. $**p < .01$.

ness, and a movement toward the "normal" on several dimensions that classically discriminate schizophrenics from normals.

These findings raise an important interpretive question: Given the pretest mismatch, is the EA improvement due to statistical artifact such as "regression to the mean" (i.e., did EAs have considerable room to improve, whereas Cs had relatively little room)? Several considerations, both logical and data-based, pertain to this issue. First, as discussed in Chapter 1 (see page 4), the modal course for the chronic schizophrenic is to languish on the back-wards with little change, particularly in his psychomotor functions (Shakow, 1962). Moreover, a common finding on the effects of psychological treatments, even with nonschizophrenics, is that the *greater* the patient's initial assets, the *greater* the likelihood that he will benefit from treatment (Luborsky, 1962; Strupp, 1962; Mogar, 1968). Thus, if there was to have been differential improvement as a function of initial status, there is a basis for expecting that initially better-functioning patients would have improved more—exactly the opposite of the present findings. This argument runs counter to the statistical regression notion and implies that the poorer initial status of EAs on the criterion performance measures should have made improvement more difficult for them.

Turning to data-based rather than logical arguments, it is necessary here to anticipate several key findings of the study. The male patient–female volunteer (MP/FV) treatment combination—the subgroup that improved most in comparison to Cs, was *not* the group most mismatched to Cs initially. Moreover, when a specially selected pretest-matched sample of EAs was compared to Cs, significant differences favoring EAs remained clearly in evidence. However, the male patients seen by male volunteers, a group that did significantly more poorly than Cs on premeasures, did not improve significantly more than Cs.

Another telling argument against a regression interpretation derives from correlational data also discussed more fully on page 102. Although initially poorer-functioning EAs were found to have improved most, initial status of Cs failed to predict clearly to change. Therefore, positive change in an initial poorly functioning group in this study was limited to Es. If the foregoing arguments have merit, a substantial portion of the EAs performance improvement is "real."

2. BEHAVIOR RATINGS

The data for within-group changes in pre–post *ward behavior* ratings revealed only a few significant changes: decreases in rated social contact and total adjustment for the male Cs, and an increase in the overall behavior rating for female Cs. Table 5.5 summarizes these results.

Table 5.6 reports changes in pre–post *group behavior* for EAs only. Comparable data were not available for Cs. In ratings of group cooperation, communication, social contact, and total adjustment, significant improvements

TABLE 5.5 *t Tests for Pre-Post Change in Ward Behavior Ratings*

	Mood[g]	Cooperation	Communication	Social contact	Total adjustment	Single overall
All EAs[a]	−1.45	−1.81	.33	−.40	−1.00	−1.47
All controls[b]	−.84	−1.25	−1.25	−.74	−1.13	.83
Male EAs[c]	−1.87	−1.49	1.34	.16	−.57	−1.86
Male controls[d]	−1.09	−.87	−1.74	−1.07*	−2.35*	−.72
Female EAs[e]	−.17	−1.08	−.71	−.76	−.84	−.22
Female controls[f]	−.16	−.59	−.52	.48	−.01	2.35*

[a] N = 150 except for overall rating, where N = 108.
[b] N = 59 except for overall rating, where N = 44.
[c] N = 86 except for overall rating, where N = 60.
[d] N = 30 except for overall rating, where N = 23.
[e] N = 64 except for overall rating, where N = 48.
[f] N = 29 except for overall rating, where N = 21.
[g] Negative t indicates a decrease in rating. $^{*}p < .05$.

were found for the total group. However, there was no significant improvement in the mood rating. The overall behavior rating improved significantly for females and for the group as a whole, but not for the male subgroup.

Thus, EAs were essentially unchanged in their ward behavior, but significantly improved in group behavior. This "discrepancy" raises the following question: Did ward personnel and college students rate the same behaviors? A partial answer is found by examining the correlations between college student and ward personnel ratings based on pre- and posttest data, i.e., the consistency across rater groups. These correlations, presented in Table 5.7, show that all six sets of ratings were positively and significantly related both for pre- and posttests. Elsewhere, the authors have discussed more fully the meaning of behavior ratings completed by different raters and administered in different situations (Rappaport & Chinsky, 1970). The median level of cross-rater and cross-situational agreement (.42) found here suggests that despite absolute discrepancies in rated behavior change, ward personnel and college students tended to judge the same patients as better adjusted.

While EAs did not show improvement on ward behavior ratings, their ratings by students, based on actual group sessions, indicated significant improvement on several dimensions: cooperation, communication, social contact, and two estimates of overall adjustment. The discrepancy between these two sets of findings may be explained either in terms of a "rater-bias" effect, or because

TABLE 5.6 *t Tests for Pre-Post Change in Group Behavior Ratings: EAs*

	Mood	Cooperation	Communication	Social contact	Total adj.	Single overall
Total E group[a]	.44	2.95**	4.46**	4.50**	3.64**	3.68**
E males[b]	– .23[d]	2.02*	3.01**	2.68**	2.13*	1.90
E females[c]	1.02	2.19*	3.42**	4.09**	3.28**	3.63**

[a]$N = 150$. [b]$N = 86$.
[c]$N = 64$. [d]Negative t indicates a decrease in rating.
*$p < .05$. **$p < .01$.

there were real differences in manifest change between the two situations upon which the ratings were based.

Intrinsic to the rater-bias interpretation, is the assumption that college students, being motivated, owing to their own ego-involvement in the project, find positive patient change, and produce positively "haloed" patient ratings. This would not be the case with attendants who neither had an expectancy for patient improvement, nor a motivation to find it, since they were not closely identified with the program. Indeed, some attendants were openly hostile to the project and not seriously incorporated into it—a point to be further developed at the end of this chapter. The rater-bias argument weighs heavily on the fact that attendants and students viewed patients from different bases of need and involvement.

However, two considerations mitigate against this argument and suggest that it can, at least partially, be discounted. First, whatever halo was operating in the student ratings was not generalized to *all* scales. Students reported *no* improvement in patient "mood" which includes 4 of the 17 rated items. Second, the independent judgment of students and attendants correlated positively and significantly for all six behavior-rating scales. Thus, the rating scales had some cross-rater and cross-situational agreement (Rappaport & Chinsky, 1970) and students, though generally more positive than attendants, did make similar relative discriminations in their patients' ratings.

A second possible explanation for the differential patient-improvement rates recorded by attendant and student judges is that there were real differences in the behaviors observed by the two sets of judges. In the actual group sessions, patients may have sensed that they were expected to act "normally" (see page 157). The group meetings were a world apart from the typical routine custodial life of the hospital patient. Thus, situational differences (Mischel, 1968, 1969) between the group meetings and the daily conditions of ward living, may have contributed to genuinely different patient behavior in those two settings. Such an interpretation is consonant with observations, both by students

TABLE 5.7 *Relations between Ward Behavior Ratings and Group Behavior Ratings*[a]

Scale (ward & group)	*r* (Pre)	*r* (Post)
Mood	.19	.32
Cooperation	.30	.36
Communication	.45	.50
Social contact	.48	.56
Total adjustment	.48	.52
Single overall	.26	.29

[a]N = 150 for all except single overall N = 108; all r's are significant $p < .01$.

and supervisors, as they watched patients returning to the ward after-the-sessions (see Chapter 7). Many patients whose group had become at least moderately outgoing and relaxed in the group, withdrew upon returning to their ward and reverted to their earlier listless, apathetic behavior.

This view is consistent, structurally, with the oft-cited separation of the "therapeutic hour" and the other 23 hours in a patient's day, and is mindful of Rotter's (1954) assertion that situational factors create specific rather than general expectancies. Put in a more behavioral framework, perhaps the contingencies maintaining disordered behavior remained unchanged on the ward, despite the group efforts. While the group situation may have encouraged better adjusted behavior, returning to the drab ward surround perhaps reinstated strong behavioral cues that more closely approached the initially established ward baseline. Interestingly, Poser (1966), whose program was similar to the present one, also failed to find significant ward behavior improvement in patients whose test performance had improved markedly. Anker and Walsh (1961) who used nonprofessionals as group leaders on the *ward* did, however, find ward-behavior improvement. Perhaps by conducting their program on the ward and by involving ward personnel, these investigators succeeded in modifying situational cues and expectancies both for attendants and patients. Ellsworth's (1968) study, cited in Section IV, B of Chapter 1, using ward personnel in treatment roles, also yielded data congruent with the latter interpretation.

B. Between-Group Comparisons of Change Scores

1. EXPERIMENTALS VERSUS CONTROLS

To test for differences in change scores between EAs and Cs, an analysis of variance for "planned comparisons" (Hays, 1966) was used. This type of analysis permits simultaneous and direct comparison among the four E conditions (male

TABLE 5.8 *Direct Comparisons between Male Patients Seen by Female Volunteers*[a] *and Male Cs*[b]

Measure	Source	*SS*	*df*	*MS*	*F*
RT 1	Treatment	534.08	1	534.08	3.50
	Error	275.04	180	152.80	
RT 2	Treatment	590.21	1	590.21	
	Error	46074.81	174	274.25	2.15
TAPS	Treatment	867.23	1	867.23	
	Error	28054.80	180	155.86	5.56*
DS	Treatment	619.07	1	619.07	
	Error	12157.20	180	67.54	9.17**
VF	Treatment	133.07	1	133.07	
	Error	3236.40	180	17.98	7.40**
Stroop A	Treatment	402.71	1	402.71	
	Error	48244.88	168	882.41	.46
Stroop B	Treatment	296.24	1	296.24	
	Error	230128.08	168	1369.81	.22
Stroop C	Treatment	21600.00	1	21600.00	
	Error	1442006.88	156	9249.98	2.34
Stroop total	Treatment	67186.24	1	67186.24	
	Error	19121.40	155	192121.40	.35
Figure ground	Treatment	3.14	1	3.14	
	Error	1006.20	180	5.59	.56
Ward mood	Treatment	1.39	1	1.39	
	Error	1998.15	173	11.55	.12
Ward cooperation	Treatment	5.57	1	5.57	
	Error	1823.42	173	10.54	.53
Ward communication	Treatment	30.49	1	30.49	
	Error	1947.98	173	11.26	2.71
Ward social contact	Treatment	82.13	1	82.13	
	Error	2354.53	173	13.61	6.05*
Total overall adj.	Treatment	309.49	1	309.49	
	Error	21057.56	173	121.72	2.54
Single overall rating	Treatment	2.10	1	2.10	
	Error	95.04	108	.88	2.39

[a]*N* varies from 31 to 19. [b]*N* varies from 31 to 19.
$^{*}p < .05$. $^{**}p < .01$.

patient–female volunteer, male patient–male volunteer, female patient–male volunteer, and female patient–female volunteer) and between E subgroups and their respective Cs.

As stated earlier (see page 93), one of the four treatment groups MP/FV improved significantly more than all others in comparison to Cs. Table 5.8 reports four significant improvements, each favoring MP/FV over C: speed of tapping, digit symbol substitution, verbal fluency, and social contact. The same directional trend, though not significant, was found with other variables: RT 1 and RT 2, Stroop Card C, and three behavior-rating scales. Table 5.9 presents mean improvement scores for MP/FVs and Cs for the performance and behavioral criterion measures. This table indicates that all significant and directional MP/FV versus C differences favored the former. Therefore, significant improvement of E males, cited earlier, may reflect the heavy contribution of the MP/FV subgroup. Other E-subgroups did not consistently demonstrate greater improvement than Cs (Rappaport, 1968).

2. PRETEST-MATCHED GROUPS

The unforeseen failure in pretest matching of Es and Cs seriously complicated the interpretation of differential group change reported in the preceding section. Therefore, a decision was made to match subgroups of EA and C on pretest scores and to repeat the change-score analyses based on these newly constituted groups. To achieve a tight match, it was necessary to reduce the EAs to 88 *S*s (22 in each of the four treatment conditions) and the Cs to 44. For these newly constituted groups, pretest mean differences were generally small and only one (Stroop Card C) reached significance (Rappaport, 1968).

Mean change-scores for matched EAs and Cs were then analyzed in the same way as for the larger EA and C groups, to test for differences between groups. As in the prior analyses involving total groups, improvement scores among the matched E and C subgroups were consistently highest in the MP/FV subgroup. When this group was compared directly with male Cs, the results were virtually the same as they had been for the larger group. Three significant differences favored MP/FVs: RT 1, speed of tapping, and digit symbol substitution, and on three other measures directionally comparable differences approached significance: RT 2, Stroop Card C, and social contact (Rappaport, 1968).

3. THE MALE PATIENT–FEMALE VOLUNTEER COMBINATION

Both of the preceding EA versus C analyses used reduced *N*s to equalize cell sizes and compared individual criterion measures. Hence, the MP/FV versus male C comparisons did not, in those analyses, use all available data. To extend these comparisons by using the largest possible *N*s, additional analyses were carried out using all *S*s in these two groups—45 MP/FV attenders and 32 comparable Cs.

Pretest differences between these two groups were examined using a discriminant function analysis which permitted comparisons to be based on a combined criterion measure, as well as on individual measures. Although some significant group differences were found on individual variables, the overall group difference, combining all variables, was not significant (Rappaport, 1968).

TABLE 5.9 *Mean Change Scores for Male Patients with Female Volunteers and Male Control Patients*

Measure	Male patient/ female volunteer	Male control
RT 1	5.06	– .81
RT 2	7.45	1.07
TAPS	1.42	–6.06
DS	5.61	– .71
VF	2.45	– .48
Stroop A	8.17	2.90
Stroop B	19.31	14.79
Stroop C	52.15	12.15
Stroop total[b]	102.12	30.23
Figure ground	1.29	.84
Ward mood	– .41	– .72
Ward cooperation	.21	– .41
Ward communication	.38	–1.66
Ward social contact	.69	–1.69
Total overall adj.	.52	–4.10
Single overall rating	.21	– .26

[a]For all measures the higher the score the greater the improvement.

[b]Since all patients could not complete all Stroop cards, Stroop total is not a simple sum of A, B, and C.

Comparison of change scores for these same groups (Table 5.10), however, yielded significant differences for five variables, as well as a significant overall difference between groups using the combined criteria. This analysis again demonstrated that the MP/FV subgroup improved significantly more than did male Cs.

Although the overall pretest discriminant function reported was not significant, it did approach significance. Accordingly, an attempt was made to match MP/FV and C subgroups even more closely on pretest scores. By dropping six Cs, based on their pretest scores, the pretest discriminant function between groups was minimized to a point indicating their clear overall comparability (Rappaport, 1968). Comparing this new pretest matched C group to the MP/FV group with respect to improvement scores yielded an overall discriminant function indicating significantly greater improvement for the latter (Rappaport, 1968).

Earlier in this chapter, we reported that significant within-group improvement was found for EA males. The preceding analyses suggest that much of this improvement was due to sharp improvement in the MP/FV subgroup. To confirm that point, a separate, but structurally similar set of comparisons was carried out contrasting the second male EA subgroup, those seen by male volunteers (MP/MV), to male Cs. Results of this analysis were quite different from those found for the MP/FV combination. Discriminant function analysis

TABLE 5.10 *Discriminant Function Analysis of Change Scores for Male Patient–Female Volunteer Group and Male Control Group*

Measure	K^d	Experimental group[a] Mean	Experimental group[a] SD	Control group[b] Mean	Control group[b] SD	F (df = 1,75)
RT 1[c]	30	33.69	9.98	29.16	4.87	5.49*
RT 2	60	64.84	17.79	60.88	8.31	1.34
TAPS	40	42.44	12.59	33.94	10.59	9.47**
DS	40	44.31	7.81	39.25	6.30	8.96**
VF	20	21.67	5.15	19.63	4.21	3.32
Stroop A	100	109.58	35.01	102.91	20.33	.91
Stroop B	80	97.20	30.80	94.81	34.30	.10
Stroop C	250	295.20	80.53	262.13	43.03	4.37*
Figure ground	10	10.93	2.73	10.97	1.97	.00
Ward mood	10	9.68	2.78	9.41	2.70	.19
Ward cooperation	10	9.88	2.49	9.63	2.40	.21
Ward communication	10	10.24	2.98	9.38	1.79	2.11
Ward social contact	20	20.84	3.41	19.03	2.43	6.41*
Single overall rate	4	3.93	.77	3.78	.93	.60
Total [e]weighted discriminant function F		F = 2.22* (df = 14, 62)				

[a]N = 45. [b]N = 32.
[c]Higher scores equal more improvement for all measures.
[d]Constants added to eliminate negative numbers.
[e]Excludes Stroop total and rating-scale total.
*p = .05. **p = .01.

showed that MP/MVs were significantly mismatched (i.e., less well-functioning than Cs) at the pretest point and that following program participation, they had not improved significantly more than the Cs (Rappaport, 1968). Thus, we conclude that the earlier demonstrated overall improvement of EA males, in comparison to Cs, was due primarily to improvement in the MP/FV subgroup.

4. SUMMARY OF OUTCOME DATA

Since the preceding sections consisted of rapid-fire presentations of a series of complex analyses of patient outcome data, a summary is in order.

Within-group change analysis for EAs and Cs indicated significant improvements mainly for the former. However, when *amount* of EA improvement, based on both the total group or pretest matched subgroups, was compared directly to amount of C-improvement, only a few, significant differences (those nonsystematic) were found to hold for *all* treatment groups. Meaningful improvement differences between EAs and Cs were clearest for male patients. In particular, the MP/FV group improved significantly more than did male Cs, both on individual test measures and on overall combinatory criterion. These results held for the raw MP/FV–male C comparison, as well as for subgroups of the two, closely matched on premeasures. The significant within-group improvement of male EAs left open the possibility that the between-group differences might also have held for male patients seen by male volunteers. However, structurally comparable analyses demonstrated that this was not the case. Thus, interpretation of significant improvement within the experimental group must be qualified to take into account the patient–volunteer sex combination. Such qualification helps to explain a seeming discrepancy between the large number of significant EA within-group improvement signs and the lack of consistent between-group differences.

Our findings in this area accord with those of Poser (1966) who also reported significant improvement in an MP/FV combination when compared with untreated male Cs. Since Poser used *only* the MP/FV treatment condition, the present data raise the possibility that his conclusions, as well as our own, may be limited to a particular student–patient treatment combination.

The striking improvement in the MP/FV group warrants further consideration. Perhaps it is not surprising that the program was generally more effective with male patients. Sanders, Smith, and Weinman (1967) found that chronic males improved more than any other of their subgroups, following socioenvironmental treatment. Ellsworth (1968) in a related program for schizophrenics, also found the greatest and most stable improvement in chronic males. Several other investigators (Cumming & Henry, 1961; Schooler, 1963) have observed that over the normal course of confinement to mental institutions, chronic male patients lose more interest in socialization than do chronic females. Perhaps then, bringing chronic male patients to social interaction groups *is* more effective in breaking up their particular pattern of hospitalization. However, in this project all male patients did not improve equally. The sex of the student group leader was an important factor in determining the extent of their improvement.

The improvement of the MP/FV subgroup cannot be attributed to different attitudes or personality characteristics of female group leaders. As will be seen in Chapter 6, female students did not differ from males on personality measures. Moreover, it was not simply the female student-leader that was the change agent, since female patients seen by female student-leaders (FP/FV) did not show markedly greater improvement than their comparable Cs. Only the particular combination of male patient and female volunteer led to effective change.

The most obvious explanation for these findings is that of rekindled patient interest in the opposite sex, triggered off by attractive, young female group-leaders. This may have brought male patients, with long histories of isolation and apathy, a significant step closer to the world of reality. A series of observations and clinical impressions (see Chapter 7) support this view. For example, some male patients who, before the program, were the epitome of poor grooming, soon began to show up for their female student leaders, clean shaven with shined shoes, and wearing ties. This interpretation is admittedly based on a combination of logic and speculation. The present findings along with Poser's (1966) earlier similar ones, point however, to the need for further study of the effectiveness of the MP/FV combination and the reasons for its effectiveness.

IV. RELATIONSHIP BETWEEN PATIENT CHARACTERISTICS AND CHANGE SCORES

The five initial-status, demographic variables obtained from hospital records and the posttest Peabody IQ scores were correlated, for EAs, with pre–post change scores on the 16 criterion measures. Since there were no significant sex differences in these correlations, a single total-group matrix is presented in Table 5.11. The correlations are generally low, only 8 of 96 reach significance. Thus, no single prestatus demographic measure predicts systematically to improvement.

Initial status on the 16 performance and behavior measures was also correlated with change scores on these same measures for the pooled EA group (see Table 5.12). Of these 256 correlations, 120 were statistically significant. Although there is some nonindependence among these 256 correlations, the number reaching significance was substantial—nearly half of the total. Of the significant correlations, 108 were negative (i.e., indicating a relationship between *poorer* initial status and improvement) and only 12 positive. Each pretest measure also correlated significantly and negatively both with change on that same measure and on at least several other relatively independent criteria. These data indicate that initially less intact EAs (defined by their preexperiment performance level) improved most after exposure to the program.

Without similar correlational data for Cs, it is difficult to know if these findings are due to the passage of time alone, the test–retest procedure, or to program effects. For this reason, a structurally similar analysis, correlating pretest and change scores, was carried out for Cs. The total of 118 of 256 significant correlations suggests that pretest status of Cs also related to change (see Table 5.13). In this case, however, 53 of the significant correlations were positive and 65 negative, indicating that *direction* of change was more complicated for Cs. Initial poor-functioning did not predict consistently to improve-

TABLE 5.11 *Demographic Status and Change Score Correlations: EAs*

Measure	Age	Length of hospitalization	Education	IQ	Paranoid/ nonparanoid[b]	Marital status[c]
RT 1[a]	.06	.05	−.01	−.14	.12	−.07
RT 2[a]	−.06	.09	−.09	−.20	.03	−.17*
TAPS	.22**	.01	.04	.12	−.10	.19*
DS	.12	.02	.14	.30**	.01	−.01
VF	.00	.09	.02	−.09	.00	−.02
Stroop A[a]	−.06	−.03	−.15	−.13	.00	−.06
Stroop B[a]	.00	.08	−.19*	−.16	−.03	−.14
Stroop C[a]	.01	.16*	−.22**	−.12	−.06	−.12
Stroop total[a]	.04	.04	−.19**	−.16	−.03	−.06
Figure ground	.06	−.12	−.07	.01	.03	.12
Ward mood	−.06	−.08	.11	.09	.00	.06
Ward cooperation	.03	−.09	.09	.07	.06	.03
Ward communication	.03	−.04	−.02	−.10	.02	.01
Ward social contact	.00	−.05	.02	−.06	.06	−.10
Total adjustment	.05	−.05	.10	.03	−.06	−.01
Single overall rating	.04	.01	.04	.08	.13	.04

[a]Log Transformations were used for all time measures in order to normalize the distributions.

[b]1 = nonparanoid; 2 = paranoid.

[c]1 = married (ever); 2 = never married.

$*p < .05$. $**p < .01$.

ment; in nearly half the cases for Cs, better initial functioning predicted to improvement. Moreover, for Cs, direction of change on a given measure was not systematically related to initial scores on that measure. For some measures, the correlation between prestatus and change was negative; for others it was positive. Thus, the high number of significant correlations between poor prestatus and improvement in EA group seems to be specifically associated with program participation.

In summary, for EAs, consistent, significant relations between demographic measures and patient improvement were not found. Improvement for EAs did, however, relate, significantly and negatively, to pretest performance scores. For Cs, there were also significant relations between pretest scores and change measures; however, the direction of these relations was inconsistent. Initial "Social-competence" (Zigler & Phillips, 1960) was unrelated to patient improvement but the adequacy-of-functioning dimension, defined by the 16 criterion premeasures, was related to patient change. Among EAs, those who initially performed most poorly improved the most.

TABLE 5.12 *Pretest and Change Score Correlations: EAs*

	Change scores															
Pretest	RT1	RT2	TAPS	DS	VF	SA	SB	SC	ST	FG	M1	M2	M3	M4	MT	OV
RT1	−.81**	−.39**	−.22**	−.25**	−.30**	−.15	−.37**	−.28**	−.39**	−.19*	.03	.03	−.02	−.17*	−.02	−.09
RT2	−.43**	−.58**	−.17*	−.16*	−.30**	−.10	−.21	−.18*	−.21**	−.12	−.07	−.16*	−.16*	−.20*	−.17*	−.08
TAPS	−.13	.00	−.39*	−.20*	−.16*	.04	−.10	−.11	−.15	−.06	.08	.18*	−.01	−.08	.07	−.10
DS	.08	−.20*	−.05	−.51**	−.29**	.08	−.08	.06	−.08	−.30**	.32**	.20*	.15	−.23**	.23**	.03
VF	.03	−.04	−.15	−.30**	−.51**	.05	−.19*	−.06	−.20*	−.25**	.13	.18*	.01	−.21**	.10	−.01
Stroop A	−.32**	−.34**	−.25**	−.05	−.03	−.19*	−.25**	−.22**	−.20*	−.09	−.25**	.08	−.15	.10	−.16*	−.24**
Stroop B	−.45**	−.37**	−.22**	−.12	−.07	−.44**	−.57**	−.57**	−.58**	−.15	−.22**	−.19*	−.13	.09	−.18*	−.17*
Stroop C	−.26**	−.07	−.18*	−.17*	−.17*	−.25**	−.52**	−.71**	−.68**	−.06	−.09	−.08	−.12	.00	−.08	−.15
Stroop total	−.42**	−.28**	−.23**	−.11	−.04	−.32**	−.54**	−.69*	−.61**	−.03	−.20*	−.16*	−.18*	.10	−.17*	−.20*
FG	.03	.17*	−.01	−.25**	−.12	.12	−.17*	.05	−.11	−.45**	−.20*	.26**	.25**	.00	−.30*	.11
MACC																
Mood (M1)	.02	−.16*	.06	.16*	.24**	.12	.09	−.04	.05	−.14	−.47**	−.18*	−.12	−.02	−.26**	−.17*
Coop. (M2)	.05	−.01	.20*	.10	.16*	.05	.07	−.03	.04	.05	−.18*	−.36**	−.03	−.07	−.20*	−.04
Comm. (M3)	−.03	.00	.06	.01	−.01	.03	−.07	−.11	−.11	.09	−.20*	−.12	−.34**	−.22**	−.25**	−.13
Soc. cont. (M4)	−.06	−.19*	.09	−.16*	−.22*	.07	−.04	.08	−.03	−.20*	.09	.15	.05	−.44**	.04	.01
Total adj. (MT)	.00	.04	.09	.08	..	.12	.02	.06	−.01	.09	−.25**	−.16*	−.13	−.20*	−.22*	−.03
Overall	.04	.07	−.21**	−.12	−.17*	−.11	−.15	−.19*	−.19*	−.08	−.03	−.03	−.15	−.11	.08	−.49**

*r of .16 < p .05. **r of .21 < p .01.

TABLE 5.13 *Pretest and Changes Score Correlations: Cs*

Pretest	Change scores															
	RT 1	RT 2	TAPS	DS	VF	SA	SB	SC	ST	FG	M1	M2	M3	M4	MT	OV
RT 1	.45**	.37**	–.09	–.39**	–.44**	.36**	–.25*	.25*	–.05	–.31*	.37**	.42**	.22	–.41**	.33*	.03
RT 2	.59**	.09	–.13	–.38**	–.32**	.27*	–.09	.07	–.14	–.29*	.34**	.37**	.18	–.39**	.29*	.00
TAPS	.09	.10	–.44**	.00	–.08	–.06	.03	–.09	–.08	.12	.14	.14	.18	.03	.13	.22
DS	.34**	.40**	–.09	–.44**	–.26*	.05	–.27*	.13	–.11	–.27*	.40**	.35**	.39**	–.30*	.37**	–.01
VF	.33**	.38**	–.04	–.28**	–.43*	.21	–.17	.15	–.04	–.26*	.18	.16	.12	–.33**	.14	.01
Stroop A (SA)	.14	.03	–.19	–.29**	–.20	–.14	–.15	.17	–.07	–.31*	.00	.13	–.15	–.33**	–.07	.05
Stroop B (SB)	–.19	–.31*	–.05	–.17	–.02	–.18	–.50**	–.14	–.30*	–.11	–.10	–.20	–.23	–.17	–.24	–.13
Stroop C (SC)	.58**	.25*	.03	–.41**	–.29+	.06	–.21	.05	–.30*	–.27*	.33**	.46**	.21	–.34**	.31*	.00
Stroop T (ST)	–.06	–.25*	–.12	–.16	–.06	–.25*	–.26*	–.32*	–.47**	.01	–.10	–.07	–.23	–.09	–.18	–.09
FG	.26*	.39**	.05	–.17	–.13	.04	–.16	.27*	.06	–.41**	.17	.17	.22	–.12	.21	.05
MACC																
Mood (M1)	–.51**	–.38**	.13	.44**	.46**	–.26*	.21	.04	.27*	.40**	–.52**	–.32*	.14	.41**	–.33*	.10
Coop. (M2)	–.34**	–.25**	.10	.40**	.43**	–.18	.17	.06	.25*	.26*	–.50**	–.51**	–.32*	.25*	–.48*	–.06
Comm. (M3)	–.39**	–.35**	.03	.42**	.54**	–.28*	.19	.00	.22	.39*	–.45**	–.39**	–.34**	.25*	–.44**	.01
Soc cont. (M4)	.48**	.42**	.0	–.26*	–.06	.08	–.17	.25*	–.04	–.17	.15	.22	.25**	–.42*	.15	–.03
Total adj. (MT)	–.39**	–.29*	.06	.45**	.55**	–.28*	.20	.07	.25*	.39**	–.54**	–.43*	–.26*	.27*	–.46**	.00
Overall	–.11	–.01	–.13	.20	32**	.00	.02	.07	.24	.26*	–.06	.02	.00	.15	–.02	–.27*

*r of $.25 < p$ .05. **r of $.33 < p$ .01.

This finding does not accord well with the observation, based primarily on treatment of less disturbed individuals, that the initially better adjusted patient profits most from treatment (Luborsky, 1962; Strupp, 1962). It is, however, consistent with recent findings based on chronic mental patients. For example, among chronic patients, Sanders *et al.* (1967) found that older males with long periods of hospitalization benefited most from a program of social interaction therapy. A similar finding was reported by Ellsworth (1968). Sanders *et al.*(1967) hypothesized that such patients have markedly reduced drive-levels, necessitating considerable stimulation for positive change to occur. However, once stimulation reaches a certain level, the likelihood of significant improvement is much greater. By contrast, more intact patients may be so involved with "inner affective pressure" that they profit less from increased social stimulation. While the specific Sanders *et al.* (1967) findings, relating age and length of hospitalization to improvement, were not replicated here, their explanation may fit other of our findings. Conceivably, patients with poor pretest functioning in our study responded more to the increased stimulation provided by college students, leading to some arousal from the slumber of institutionalism.

V. PATIENT PERCEPTIONS OF THE COLLEGE STUDENTS

A. Item Analysis

Responses to the 25-item PEP scale were analyzed in several ways. The general negative view that mental patients had of college students before the experiment started, was reported in Chapter 4. Following patient assignments to E and C groups, pretest responses of these two groups were compared, individually for each item, using 2 X 2 contingency tables (Siegel, 1956), to test for possible differences between groups in their initial perceptions of physicians and college students. The two groups did not differ on a single item at pretest (Rappaport, 1968). Structurally, comparable posttest analyses (Rappaport, 1968) indicated five significant differences between groups. Proportionally more Es than Cs saw college students as more giving of advice and gentle and less critical, hard to please, and bossy. Collectively, these findings indicate a positive shift in Es' perceptions of college students by the end of the program.

Each item was also analyzed separately for Es and Cs for changes in frequency of endorsement of doctors versus college students from pre- to posttest. For each group, the expected postendorsement frequency, by item, for doctor or college student, was established by its own pretest frequency (corrected for slight posttest decreases in number). Table 5.14 indicates that Es shifted significantly toward more favorable views of college students on 18 of the 25 items. Thus, on the posttest, significantly more Es described college students as more likely than doctors to give advice, sense their feelings, and give encouragement. They also described college students as more likely to be calm, sympathetic, gentle, considerate, interested in them, eager to help them, like themselves, fun to be with, and liking them and liking to be with them. In addition, significantly fewer Es saw college students as critical, blunt, hardworking, hard to please, and bossy.

For Cs, there were only four such significant changes on the posttest. These increases were toward stronger endorsement of college students on the items: sensing your feelings, calm, giving of encouragement, and eager to help.

TABLE 5.14 *E and C Group χ^2's for Change in Frequency of Endorsement of College Students on PEP Items*

Item no.[a]	E group χ^2	C group χ^2
1	18.98***[b]	2.35
2	.24	1.73
3	13.02***[c]	.36
4	18.79***[b]	10.48**[b]
5	22.36***[b]	6.00*[b]
6	4.56*[c]	2.51
7	31.95***[b]	7.51**[b]
8	.22	.89
9	3.01	.17
10	3.77	.29
11	6.06*[c]	1.04
12	10.56***[c]	.50
13	23.87***[b]	.58
14	3.48	2.96
15	18.16***[c]	.13
16	34.44***[b]	.13
17	33.96***[b]	2.77
18	.39	1.43
19	1.92	.01
20	22.01***[b]	1.94
21	27.71***[b]	4.01*[b]
22	5.01*[b]	.01
23	6.63*[b]	2.77
24	15.26***[b]	1.14
25	6.09*[b]	.12

[a]Items appear in Table 4.6.

[b]Change in direction of more endorsement of college students.

[c]Change in direction of less endorsement of college students.

$*p < .05$. $**p < .01$. $***p < .001$.

On each of these items, the expected cell frequency for college students was less than 10, increasing the probability that relatively small changes in observed frequencies would be statistically significant. However, even including these four changes, Cs were stable on most items, whereas Es showed a markedly more favorable attitude to college students.

B. Cluster Analysis

In order to evaluate global changes in patient perception of students, the first 18 items of the PEP were grouped for analysis according to Apfelbaum's (1958) clusters: nurturant, model, and critic (six items per cluster). Cluster scores were obtained by summing, for individual patients, the frequency of endorsement for *college students* across all items within each cluster. Each cluster had a potential range of scores from 0 to 6.

For these analyses, EAs were compared to Cs under the expectation that changes in perceptions would result from differential contact with students. The three cluster scores were analyzed for change, by group, from pre- to posttest, using a 2 X 2 analysis of variance for repeated measures. Table 5.15 reports group means and analyses of variance for the nurturant and critic clusters. The significant Treatment X Time interaction reflects an increase among EAs, but not Cs, in the perception of students as nurturant in comparison to physicians. Table 5.15 also shows a nonsignificant trend among EAs, but not Cs, in the perception of college students as less critical. Structurally similar analyses for the model cluster failed to reveal significant group differences.

One explanation for the seeming effectiveness of nonprofessional mental health workers is that patients see them as closer to themselves in the "social hierarchy" than professionals (Rioch, 1966), thereby facilitating development of meaningful interpersonal relationships. Cowen (1967), proposes that this factor may be a "central element in a variety of helping approaches, for example 'AA' ... Recovery Incorporated ... or Synanon ... where efforts are made to reduce the social distance factors ... [p. 428]." Even before contact with students was established, chronic patients saw them, more than physicians, as: "like themselves" and "fun to be with," items suggesting less perceived social distance between patient and student (see Chapter 4). While Cs perception of college students were stable over time, Es increasingly saw students as nurturant.

This finding takes on greater significance if one considers the test instrument used to assess patient perceptions. In order to endorse college students positively, patients *had* to respond negatively to physicians. During the testing sessions, some patients expressed concern about this clear-cut choice, particularly so, since they were tested by people whom they considered to be hospital personnel. Despite this potential source of anxiety, many patients responded

TABLE 5.15 *Analysis of Variance for Change in Patient's Endorsement of College Students as Nurturant and Critic*

Nurturant	*SS*	*df*	*MS*	*F*
A (treatment)	11.4	1	11.41	4.91**
B (time, pre-post)	31.68	1	31.68	20.63****
A X B	9.68	1	9.68	6.31***
Error	244.13	159	1.54	
Critic				
A (treatment)	32.09	1	32.09	12.77***
B (time, pre-post)	15.21	1	15.21	8.67**
A X B	4.58	1	4.58	2.61
Error	279.20	159	1.76	

Mean Scores

	Nurturant		Critic	
	Pre	*Post*	*Pre*	*Post*
EA	1.33	2.20	2.65	2.05
C	1.30	1.43	3.08	2.98

$^{**}p < .02$. $^{**}p < .01$. $^{***}p < .001$.

more favorably to students on the posttest. Evidently, they felt sufficiently positive about their relationship to a college student to be able to express this change in view, even though it may have produced anxiety to do so.

Prior studies have shown positive attitude changes toward mental patients on the part of students who had participated in volunteer programs (Scheibe, 1965; Turner, Holzberg, & Knapp, 1967). Similar attitude changes were found in this program (see Chapter 6). Less frequently demonstrated, however, is change in patients' perceptions. That such change took place in chronic hospitalized schizophrenics is of significance in thinking about tertiary prevention programs. The finding suggests that patients are indeed capable of forming meaningful interpersonal relationships—an interesting one when viewed against the widespread belief that chronic schizophrenics are largely incapable of so doing (e.g., Noyes & Kolb, 1958).

Perhaps long-held notions about the schizophrenic's inability to relate meaningfully to others derive from the mental health professional's typical interactions with such patients and the context of those interactions. However, in this study students were enthusiastic, energetic, hopeful, and unencumbered by absolute knowledge or unshakable pessimism. They approached the situation with the naive expectation that they would be relating to other human beings. From the patients' standpoint, college students were seen initially as "like themselves," a view that crystallized even further during the course of the program. Perhaps, it *is* easier for many patients to relate to college students than to professionals; or, as Guerney (1969) has observed, for some patients, nonprofessionals may be more important than professionals as "social reinforcers."

VI. FOLLOW-UP STUDY

Follow-up possibilities were limited by the departure of the first two authors at the end of the project. These authors had been attached to the Rochester State staff throughout the duration of the program. Nevertheless, since we were interested in longer term, as well as immediate project effects, a limited file follow-up was initiated about a year after the study had ended to determine the status of all patient participants. Data collection was carried out by two undergraduates who spent considerable time researching as many patients as possible and abstracting progress notes from their charts. The main categories recorded were *change-in-status* indices such as: "discharge," "assignment to family or convalescent care," "ward reassignment," "change in voluntary–involuntary status," and "assignment to rehabilitation"—*job status; physicians' progress notes* (based on periodic patient reexamination and reevaluation); and *changes in medication.* Collectively, after abstracting, such materials never exceeded one page per patient.

A file search over a period of several months, turned up data for 300 of the original 320 E and C patients. Of the 20 we were unable to include in the follow-up, six were known to have died; the remainder were assumed dead or, their records were assumed to be misplaced at times of ward transfer. Specifically, we were able to locate 157 of the 161 EAs, 85 of the 95 ENAs, and 58 of the 64 Cs. We were most successful in locating EAs and least successful in locating ENAs—a finding reminiscent of the performance posttest data, when most "fails" were ENAs.

A 7-point rating scale was constructed to evaluate the file data and to render a follow-up judgment of "current status." The points of the scale were defined as follows:

- −1 Patient has become worse.
- 0 No improvement.
- +1 Slight improvement (improvement on one factor studied).
- +2 Moderate improvement (improvement on two factors studied).
- +3 Considerable improvement (improvement of three or four factors studied).
- +4 Sufficiently improved to be placed on convalescent or family care.
- +5 Discharged.

Ratings based on the file data were made independently by a psychologist and an undergraduate psychology student. Interrater reliability was .71. Of particular interest is the finding that only 10% of the patients were rated in either the +4 or +5 categories; this fact can be read as an indication either of limited program effectiveness or of the hospital's reluctance to modify patient status.

Mean improvement scores for the three groups were as follows: EA = 1.06, ENA = .39, C = .22. The difference between EAs and Cs reached statistical significance ($t = 2.16$; $p > .05$). Some positive program effects remained in evidence a year after the study had ended. On the other hand, it is discouraging to note that the absolute improvement level of EAs was only slight and that such a small percentage of the *total* patient group had graduated to family or convalescent care or discharge. Once again, the data point to the extreme difficulties of reversing deeply entrenched pathological processes, and to the importance of better coordinating discharge policies and community resources with in-hospital treatment programs (Rappaport & Chinsky, 1970).

VII. SOME GENERAL OBSERVATIONS

Most patients in our study had experienced long-term institutionalization and had presumably suffered many of its detrimental effects (Goffman, 1961). Similarly, the institution itself may be viewed as a product of its long-term custodial philosophy. The activities in which hospital residents—both staff and patients—have typically engaged mirror this philosophy. One way to assess the impact of college-student volunteer groups is by their effect on on-going hospital programs and activities, which reflect changes in the hospital as a social system. As recently as the summer before this program started, prospects were poor for developing a large-scale intervention for chronic patients at Rochester State Hospital. The characteristic problems of large state hospitals, particularly manpower shortages, precluded such programming (see Chapter 2). When the pilot study was undertaken at Rochester State, the likelihood of large-scale use of college students as patient group leaders was still limited. Indeed, there was considerable staff anxiety at that time about the pilot program. It would have been difficult to predict, given this initial climate, that by the end of the program, several responsible hospital administrators would formally request continuation of the program. These requests reflect at least a token move toward a more active concern in patient care. The program is continuing at Rochester State.

A disappointing shortcoming of the program was its failure to have sufficiently and meaningfully incorporated ward attendants and, thus, its failure to have substantially changed their attitudes. The importance of genuine attendant involvement is central to a program of this type (see page 86, where the role of ward personnel was considered in detail). In retrospect, it would be appropriate to include ward attendants in the planning stages and have them become an integral part of the program. An alternative directed to the same problem is to use nonprofessionals in actual on-the-ward groups, hopefully to effect meaningful, enduring change in expectancies for ward behavior rather than simply for encapsulated group meetings. The need for greater involvement of regular hospital staff *together* with imaginative use of nonprofessionals seem clear, particularly if the present findings are considered alongside the impressive results reported by Ellsworth (1968).

The possibility that under-involvement of ward personnel was a limiting factor in the present investigation, gave rise to a further smaller-scale study at Rochester State Hospital during the year following this project (Mace, 1969). This second research bears consideration here, both because it follows logically from the major study and because it is pertinent to the issue under discussion. Mace, as did the present investigators, built his investigation around college-student volunteers working with patient groups. However, he restricted his E groups to some variant of the MP/FV combination, which we found effective. His target group again consisted of chronic schizophrenics; indeed, in terms of bellweather criteria of chronicity such as mean age and length of hospitalization, if anything, it was even *more* chronic than was our sample. Mace's evaluation battery, though similar to the present one, used fewer performance tests and a larger number of actual behavioral ratings. The number of his patients, both E and C, was about 25% of the present samples.

The most important difference between Mace's study and this one, involves his more extensive and effective use of ward personnel with the several patient subgroups. In all, Mace used three E-conditions, each with three subgroups, built around a nucleus of a female student leader and 6–8 patients. His first class of E subgroups included one female student leader plus eight patients. In his second, and most critical type of E group, both actual planning of program and the ways the groups would be conducted, were the joint responsibility of one female student and one male ward attendant (replicated three times for the three subgroups in this condition). Thus, student and attendant jointly led patient groups, had postmeeting contact and provided feedback to each other and participated in discussion–supervisory meetings with the program consultant. The third set of E groups was jointly led by two students, one male and one female. This was done to control the factor of male–female group leadership and the additional opportunities joint leadership provided for feedback and leader discussion. A fourth matched, no-treatment control group was included in his study.

Mace's findings though clear in their own right, did not parallel those of the present investigation in specific detail. Overall, his pooled E-groups improved more than did his C group. However, the major patient improvements were found on measures of ward behavior rather than performance test change. Together, the dual-leadership groups fared better than did the groups led by female students alone. Directionally, the female-student-plus-attendant combination, did best of all. These objective data were buttressed by observations and clinical data suggesting that the most widespread and generalized positive effects of the program came from the situation in which ward attendants had a genuine stake both in planning and implementing it. Mace's findings support the view that the positive effects of college-student volunteer programs with chronic hospitalized patients can be extended and strengthened through meaningful attendant participation.

VIII. SUMMARY

The major aim of the patient section of the study was to answer three questions about the use of nonprofessionals as helping agents in a state hospital setting. In regard to the first question, "Is this type of intervention effective?", only a qualified affirmative answer can be given. Although there is evidence of program effectiveness, this was largely due to *one* of the four treatment combinations—the MP/FV group which clearly improved more than comparable Cs.

The second question, "What are the characteristics of patients who benefit from such an intervention?" was approached in two ways. Demographic predictor measures of "social competence" (Zigler & Phillips, 1960) bore no relationship to patient improvement. However, using pretest performance and behavior indices as outcome predictors, patients who were functioning most poorly initially were found to have profitted most from the program.

The final question, "How do patients perceive college students and how do such perceptions change as a result of the program?" was answered in some detail. Initially, students were seen as more critical and less nurturant than physicians. However, they were also seen as closer to the patients in perceived "social distance." At the end of the program, patient participants came to see students significantly more favorably than initially, and more favorably, in the absolute sense, than they saw doctors. These data suggest that chronic schizophrenics *can* form meaningful interpersonal relationships, and as such, have implications for future programs in tertiary prevention.

Chapter 6

RESEARCH EVALUATION: COLLEGE STUDENTS

This chapter presents findings in four principal areas dealing with the student program leaders. Briefly, these areas are:

(1) What relationships are there between student personality attributes and patient change?
(2) How do student leaders compare with nonvolunteer controls with respect to personality variables?
(3) What attitude changes occur in student leaders as a result of program participation?
(4) How do group activities relate to initially measured student personality and attitudes as well as to patient change?

Following the procedure used in the last chapter, we shall present findings in descriptive-narrative form, based on more technical data summaries and statistical analyses.

I. STUDENT PERSONALITY AND PATIENT OUTCOME

The seemingly straightforward aim of this portion of the study was to identify the attributes of the effective student leader. However, to do so required a more precise definition of the key word, "effective," that is, specific identification of changes in patient status that operationalize the term. At the outset, this seemed to be a simple step, but certain "casualties of design" made it far more complex than originally anticipated. Initially, the plan was to use an overall group-change index, by averaging pre- to posttest change scores on the criterion measures for the eight patients comprising each subgroup. These group change scores were then to have been related to each of the student personality variables.

Two practical problems, neither anticipated beforehand, undermined this strategy. The first, noted in Chapter 5, was the mismatch of patient groups on the pretest performance measures. In terms of the concept of average improvement scores, this mismatch meant that each group had started at a different level of intactness as reflected by the criterion battery. This fact raised the question as to whether comparable absolute mean changes had the same meaning across patient groups. The second problem arose from the attendance data. As reported in Chapter 5, a patient was arbitrarily defined as a program participant if he attended two-thirds or more of his group's scheduled meetings. Had patient attrition been even across subgroups, severe problems would not have been posed for the present analyses. In fact, attrition rates were uneven across groups. Some, for example, finished with their full initial complement of eight patients, while shrinkage in one or two instances reduced the initial group to only two or three patients. Thus, average group change scores were relatively stable for groups with eight patients and quite unstable for groups with only two. Phrased otherwise, differential attrition meant that a group change score for eight patients would receive no more weight than a structurally similar, but considerably less stable score for a group of two or three.

Nevertheless, group change or improvement was at the heart of this analysis, and it had to be used in one form or another. Hence, concerted effort was made to minimize the effects of the two confounding factors just noted. This led to the development of two types of group improvement scores. The *mean improvement method* consisted simply of subtracting pretest mean group scores from posttest mean group scores and obtaining a "raw" group-difference score. Since scores on timed tests, that is, the two RT and four Stroop measures, were highly skewed because many patients took a relatively long time to complete them, pre–post change scores for these measures were based on a normalizing logarithmic transformation of the original raw-scores.

Student ratings of patient behavior in the groups were not included with the change criteria, since these ratings were potentially affected by the same student characteristics to which they were to be compared and, as such, were not "independent." Thus, 15 patient change scores, 10 performance, and five ward behavior measures (each described in Chapter 4), were used as the change criteria. Changes on the 10 performance measures were converted to standard (z) scores and added across measures to obtain a sixteenth score—a single overall performance change score for each subgroup.

The second method for assessing patient change consisted of computing *average percentage of improvement* scores for each group. Improvement from pre- to posttest, regardless of its magnitude, was given a score of 1 for each measure. A group improvement score was obtained by dividing the number of "improved" patients by the total number of patients in the group. An overall performance score was obtained by adding across the 10 performance criterion measures, as was done for the mean-change method. The percentage of improvement score does not overcome the problem of disparate group size, but it minimizes the absolute magnitude of change scores and thereby somewhat circumvents the problem of initially mismatched subgroups.

These two improvement scores yielded relatively high intercorrelations ranging from .60 to .84 for the separate measures, with a median correlation of .70. Because of these relatively high correlations between the methods and the comparable findings obtained using them as criteria, the group mean-change score was adopted as the basic criterion for most substantive analyses of relations between student attributes and patient change. Average percentage of improvement scores were utilized in a few specific instances when they offered further data clarification. In establishing the group mean change as the basis for evaluating the "effectiveness" of student leaders, it was possible to relate directly student personality variables to patient outcome indices. In the sections to follow, the results of these analyses are reported. We shall begin with the Truax and Carkhuff, A–B, and GAIT measures of talent and style.

A. Truax–Carkhuff Measures

1. RELIABILITY AND INTERSCALE CORRELATIONS AMONG TRUAX SCALES

Interrater reliabilities for the accurate empathy, nonpossessive warmth, and congruence scales were .47, .91, and .89, respectively. These correlations accord well with earlier findings (Truax & Carkhuff, 1967). Warmth and congruence intercorrelated significantly (r = .53, p = .05). However, the correlations between accurate empathy and both warmth (r = .21) and congruence (r = .04) were not statistically significant. The latter finding is inconsistent with past studies, which show relatively high interrelations among all three scales (Truax & Carkhuff, 1967) and suggests that these three measures were relatively independent in the present study.

2. CORRELATIONS OF THE TRUAX SCALES WITH OUTCOME

A series of correlations was computed (Chinsky, 1968) between the Truax measures of accurate empathy, nonpossessive warmth, and congruence and group mean change scores for the 10 individual performance measures and the overall performance change score. None of the Truax measures related significantly to improvement in performance. Intercorrelations between Truax measures and ward behavior change were also analyzed and yielded similarly negative results (Chinsky, 1968).

B. A–B Scale and Outcome

Relations between the A–B Scale, scored for A, and performance change were studied (Chinsky, 1968). Since the A–B scale was standardized on a male sample (Betz, 1962), data for the total E-group and males alone were analyzed separately. For the total group, A-scores correlated significantly with RT 1 ($r = .39$, $p = .05$). Male A-scores correlated significantly with the Stroop total, an overall measure of perceptual functioning ($r = .51$, $p = .05$). None of the r's between the A-scores and ward behavior change were significant either for the total group or for male student leaders alone (Chinsky, 1968).

C. GAIT Measures

1. RELIABILITY AND INTERSCALE CORRELATIONS: GAIT

Reliability estimates of the GAIT scales, summarized in Table 6.1, were computed using all 48 students who participated in the seminar–practicum course. Split-half reliability for student peer ratings on each of the nine individual GAIT scales and therapeutic talent (sum of the warmth, openness, and understanding scales) were computed by dividing the student raters into two groups. Column 1 of Table 6.1 presents these interrater reliabilities which ranged from .41 (accepting-warm) to .71 (quiet), with a median of .62, when corrected by the Spearman–Brown formula.

The GAIT ratings of the graduate-student observers were also intercorrelated. These observer correlations were converted to z scores (McNemar, 1962). Average correlations for the GAIT measures derived from this procedure, are presented in Column 2 of Table 6.1. The lowest observer agreement was on the "relaxed" dimension ($r = .19$), the highest on accepting-warm ($r = .64$), and the median was .48. Intercorrelations between students and observers on the 10 GAIT measures were moderate, ranging from .30 to 59 with a median of .48. These are presented in Column 3 of Table 6.1.

Intercorrelations among the GAIT subscales, based on combined observer and student ratings, were also computed to determine interscale consistency. These correlations, summarized in Table 6.2, ranged from −.02 (open and blue) to .81 (best counselor and therapeutic talent). Correlations between therapeutic talent and its three components—understanding, open, and warm—are spuriously

TABLE 6.1 *Interrater Reliability of Observer and Peer GAIT Ratings*[a]

	Measure	Peer[b]	Observer[c]	Observer/Peer
1.	Understanding	.70	.49	.32
2.	Blue	.66	.46	.49
3.	Open	.56	.42	.49
4.	Quiet	.71	.34	.48
5.	Warm	.41	.64	.53
6.	Rigid	.63	.50	.41
7.	Relaxed	.58	.19	.37
8.	Meaningful	.43	.43	.59
9.	Best counselor	.63	.40	.30
10.	Therapeutic talent	.61	.57	.45

[a]$N = 48$.
[b]Corrected by Spearman–Brown formula.
[c]Average reliability.

inflated. Each of the latter three scales, however, correlated significantly with the more independent "best counselor" rating. The rigid scale correlated significantly and negatively with each of these same three measures. The blue and quiet scales correlated positively with each other, but not with any other dimension.

GAIT reliabilities, computed separately for peers and observers as well as between peers and observers, were spotty. While many were satisfactory, a few were sufficiently low to raise serious question about the scale's usefulness. However, the interscale correlations found in this study closely replicated Goodman's (1965) earlier findings, using only male students. The comparable overall findings of the two studies, and the lack of significant sex differences in this investigation, suggest that the GAIT is about as reliable and internally consistent for females as for males.

2. CORRELATION OF THE GAIT WITH OUTCOME

Correlations were computed between combined peer and observer ratings for each GAIT measure and group mean improvement scores on the performance measures (Chinsky, 1968). Only eight of these 110 correlations were statistically significant—a number predictable by chance. Similar negative findings were obtained using both peer and observer's ratings separately as the GAIT criteria (Chinsky, 1968). Correlations between the 10 combined peer and observer ratings and the five ward behavior ratings were also examined. Only one of the 50 correlations in this matrix was significant (Chinsky, 1968). Essentially the same results were obtained using peer or observers' ratings alone as the GAIT criterion.

TABLE 6.2 *Intercorrelation of Combined Ratings on 10 GAIT Measures*

	Variable	Understanding	Blue	Open	Quiet	Warm	Rigid	Relaxed	Meaningful	Best counselor
1.	Understanding									
2.	Blue	−.31*								
3.	Open	.43**	−.02							
4.	Quiet	−.17	.61**	−.08						
5.	Warm	.59**	−.09	.63**	.15					
6.	Rigid	−.28*	−.17	−.45**	−.33*	−.70**				
7.	Relaxed	.42**	−.46**	.39**	−.16	.51**	−.24			
8.	Meaningful	.27	.25	.78**	.13	.56**	−.57**	.16		
9.	Best counselor	.76**	−.30*	.57**	−.12	.71**	−.49**	.54**	.52**	
10.	Therapeutic talent	.81**	−.17	.82**	−.04	.89**	−.57**	.53**	.64**	.81**

$^{*}p < .05$. $^{**}p < .01$.

Correlations between GAIT measures and ward behavior were also computed using average percentage of improvement scores. Table 6.3 presents these correlations for observers, peers, and combined observers and peers, respectively. Although these 150 correlations are not entirely independent, the total of 16 significant correlations exceeds chance ($\chi^2 = 10.13$, $p = .01$). As a partial control for nonindependence, one can use the eight significant correlations obtained from the structurally comparable and equally nonindependent analysis based on group mean improvement scores. Using this as a baseline, the observed number of significances in the new analysis still exceeds chance ($\chi^2 = 8.45$, $p = .01$). Nine of the 16 significant correlations involve positive relations between therapeutic talent or its components of warmth and understanding—the variables governing the initial choice of the GAIT as a predictor measure—and ward improvement. Thus, using average percentage of improvement, a weak relation is demonstrated between GAIT therapeutic effectiveness and ward behavior improvement scores in patients.

Several additional analyses using both average percentage of improvement scores and group mean improvement scores, were carried out in an attempt to minimize the effects of prescore variability and uneven subgroup size. With respect to the former, subgroups with extreme prescores were eliminated. To control for the latter, only subgroups with final patient *N*s of four or more were used. Each of these analyses yielded results comparable to those obtained using all 30 groups.

D. Interrelations among Talent Measures

The absence of robust relations between student style and talent measures and patient improvement scores prompted examination of the interrelationships among the talent measures themselves. A series of correlations were computed based on the three Truax–Carkhuff scores, A–B score, and scores on the GAIT measures (Chinsky, 1968). None of these 15 correlations approached statistical significance thus raising serious question about the extent to which they reflect anything that approximates a unitary talent measure in the present sample. Notwithstanding similarity of scale labeling (e.g., GAIT: "warm" versus Truax–Carkhuff: "nonpossessive warmth"), these measures have apparently tapped relatively independent attributes in this sample.

E. Other Personality and Attitude Measures

While predicting the attributes of the effective volunteer was most directly evaluated using the talent and style measures reported in the preceding sections, other student personality and attitude measures from the massive initial battery

TABLE 6.3 *Correlation of Observer, Peer, and Combined GAIT Ratings with Mean Percentage of Improvement Scores: Behavior Measures*

Ward outcome measure	GAIT measure									
	Understanding	Blue	Open	Quiet	Warm	Rigid	Relaxed	Meaningful	Best counselor	Therapeutic talent
					Observer					
Mood	.48**	.01	.09	.05	.39*	−.25	.14	.19	.49**	.38*
Cooperation	.14	.03	.07	.22	.41*	−.28	.05	.07	.35	.24
Communication	−.24	.13	−.13	.03	.13	−.32	.04	−.03	.07	−.10
Social contact	.19	−.24	.16	.12	.25	−.07	−.02	.17	.29	.23
Total adjustment	.23	−.12	.05	.16	.46**	−.26	.27	.04	.42*	.28
					Peer					
Mood	.27	−.01	.20	.22	.27	−.21	.10	.26	.25	.29
Cooperation	.07	.11	.15	.37*	.17	−.19	.18	.23	.09	.15
Communication	−.15	.27	−.06	.18	−.09	−.21	−.21	.05	−.13	−.12
Social contact	.18	.07	.24	−.06	.26	−.57**	.04	.20	.17	.26
Total adjustment	.10	.10	.25	.17	.22	−.26	.14	.21	.18	.22
					Combined (Peer and Observer)					
Mood	.36*	−.01	.18	.19	.38*	−.27	.13	.23	.43*	.37*
Cooperation	.10	.10	.14	.37*	.32	−.26	.17	.17	.23	.22
Communication	−.29	.20	−.11	.16	.00	−.30	−.18	.02	.07	−.16
Social contact	.11	.00	.24	−.02	.30	−.49**	.03	.22	.27	.25
Total adjustment	.12	.06	.19	.18	.37*	−.31	.21	.14	.34	.27

*$p < .05$. **$p < .01$.

provided a basis for a second, more empirical approach to the same question. Accordingly, the 49 scales derived from the PRF, ACL (self), I-E, Chapin, Self Disclosure, and Wrightsman tests were used as predictors. Data on these measures were available for the 61 *S*s from SC II plus 14 other practicum students assigned to elementary school programs. Scores of this group of 75 *S*s were factor analyzed in an effort to identify clusters of common elements within the relatively heterogeneous test battery. The first 10 derived factors, accounting for 73% of the total variance, were rotated, yielding six new factors accounting for 60% of the variance. Table 6.4 presents these six factors with descriptive labels, the amount of variance accounted for by each, specific items comprising the factors, and item-loadings.

The first and largest factor, labeled *positive versus negative self-concept,* included 12 ACL scales and PRF affiliation. The second factor consisting exclusively of 10 ACL items was an *active–passive* dimension, while the third, labeled *impulsivity–order* included six PRF scales and three ACL items. Factor IV, *autonomy* was made up of four PRF scales and the Wrightsman measure of individual differences. A fifth factor, made up of four PRF scales and one ACL item was labeled *defensiveness,* and the sixth, consisting of four PRF scales, was labeled *nonassertive independence*.

Having identified a consistent factorial structure for the test battery, the next step was to compute factor scores (e.g., autonomy, defensiveness, etc.) for each of the student leaders. To do this, *S*s scores on each item were converted to standard *z* scores, which were summed for all items comprising a given factor. This yielded a total factor score. The six resultant factor scores were correlated with patient change scores, as a further test of the relation between student personality variables and patient outcome. The number of significant correlations between these factor scores and patient change scores on the eleven test performance and five ward-behavior measures failed to exceed chance expectancy (Chinsky, 1968).

F. Prediction Data: Discussion

Substantive findings in this area failed to demonstrate stable relations between student personality and attitude measures, used as predictors, and patient change. Shortcomings of experimental design that may have contributed to this failure and the one subarea in which several positive findings were identified are considered in this section.

We can identify several methodological limitations of the study that may have diluted relations between student attributes and outcome indices. Among the most serious, is the nature of the student sample in the study. The use of a group-contact format in the program sharply restricted the size of the student sample, even though the patient *N* was sizable. The size of the patient groups

TABLE 6.4 *Factors Derived from Factor Analysis cf 49 Personality Scales*[a]

Factor I (self-concept)		Factor II (active-passive)		Factor III (impulsivity-order)	
Variable	Loading	Variable	Loading	Variable	Loading
ACL—Nurturance	−.875	ACL—Dominance	−.841	PRF—Impulsivity	−.801
ACL—Unfavorable	.871	ACL—Self-confidence	−.834	PRF—Order	.772
ACL—Affiliation	−.871	ACL—Deference	.799	PRF—Cognitive structure	.740
ACL—Personal adjustment	−.849	ACL—Abasement	.791	ACL—Order	.724
ACL—Favorable	−.777	ACL—Achievement	−.732	PRF—Play	−.556
ACL—Intraception	−.752	ACL—Autonomy	−.638	PRF—Change	−.512
ACL—Aggression	.614	ACL—Aggression	−.613	ACL—Endurance	.512
ACL—Heterosexuality	−.587	ACL—Exhibition	−.611	ACL—Liability	−.447
ACL—Autonomy	.537	ACL—Change	−.575	PRF—Social Desirability	.441
ACL—Endurance	−.518	ACL—Succorance	−.453		
ACL—Self-control	−.501				
PRF—Affiliation	−.451				
ACL—Defensiveness	−.450				
Factor IV (autonomy)		**Factor V (defensiveness)**		**Factor VI (nonassertive independence)**	
Variable	Loading	Variable	Loading	Variable	Loading
PRF—Autonomy	.780	PRF—Abasement	−.651	PRF—Aggression	−.753
PRF—Succorance	−.649	PRF—Achievement	−.558	PRF—Domiance	−.697
PRF—Social recognition	−.628	ACL—Defensiveness	.473	PRF—Dependence	−.638
PRF—Harm avoidance	−.528	PRF—Endurance	−.470	PRF—Exhibition	−.429
Wrightsman individual diff.	−.435	PRF—Nurturance	−.452		

[a] $N = 75$: 61 SC II and 14 undergraduate practicum students.

was set at eight anticipating attrition, which was, in fact, substantial. To have had more than 30 groups of this size would have exceeded the physical limits (e.g., number of available meeting rooms) of the hospital.

The total number of patients meeting the selection criteria, and the resources of project staff to provide program coordination, supervision, and consultation were also limiting factors. This restriction on the number of students in the program effectively reduced student sample size along one salient dimension to 30, rather than the seemingly substantial patient sample ($N = 161$).

Groups were carefully and successfully matched on a series of demographic factors, on the assumption that pretest performance scores would also be comparable. As discussed earlier, this was not, in fact, the case. Specific subgroups had different baselines and different levels of functioning when the study started. These initial discrepancies, in effect, became "noise" in the test of relations between student attributes and outcome scores. It would have been much more straightforward to have been able to do these analyses with all subgroups starting from a comparable performance and behavioral base.

Also discussed earlier was the fact that overall patient attrition and differential attrition for subgroups were not predictable beforehand. Thus, changes in two-patient groups using this method, unfortunately carried the same weight as changes in eight. Since group change was the prime criterion by which volunteer effectiveness was to be evaluated, a test of this relationship between these two variables was seriously weakened by very real, but noncontrollable, elements in the study.

Each of the preceding factors added error variance, or "noise," to evaluation of this basic hypothesis. Although an effort was made to cope with these problems by analyses eliminating groups decimated by attrition or extreme prescore "outlyers," such attempts were thwarted by the omnipresence of the two methodological difficulties and by the fact that substantial reduction of volunteer N could not be supported because of the initially small volunteer sample.

In retrospect, it is easier to describe preconditions that allow for a more appropriate test of the relation between student attributes and indices of patient improvement. Almost certainly, these should include more subgroups and large enough patient groups, carefully prematched on both demographic *and* test measures, to be stable even after patient dropout.

A further unexpected source of difficulty in evaluating the hypothesis under discussion, was the lack of communality among the talent and style measures derived from the Truax–Carkhuff, A–B, and GAIT. None of the correlations among these measures of presumably related attributes approached statistical significance. While this may in part reflect the restricted student sample, it also mirrors weaknesses in current techniques of personality assessment. Similarly labeled measures, presumed to tap related qualities, did not relate to each other in this study. This finding raises question as to whether these scales measure what they purport to measure (Rappaport & Chinsky, 1971).

Several other elements in the structure of the study mitigated against finding relations between student attributes and patient improvement scores. A concern illustrating this observation grows out of the question: "What factors, other than student personality, could have influenced patient change?" One of the most important of these potentially was patient reaction to the program itself, which was unique and novel at Rochester State. Some patients had had no contact whatsoever with an "interested" person from outside the hospital in several years. The patient groups began with little forewarning and, for some patients, a marked change in daily routine occurred. The introduction of this new experience may, by itself, have been a potentially telling change-agent independent of student personality or attitude factors. By analogy, the alcoholic, suffering acute withdrawal symptoms, cares very little if his next drink is Calverts or Canadian Club. A further extension of the argument that variables intrinsic to the study, other than student personality characteristics, were potentially significant change agents is found in the datum that the most improved of the four E subgroups, was the MP/FV group. Consideration of this finding already offered in Chapter 5, led us to conclude that student *personality* attributes were not prime casual agents of such change.

Another attribute of the study that reduced the likelihood of finding relations between student leader attributes and patient change was the group approach. The group format dilutes the student's specific personal impact, since he is but one of many persons interacting in the situation.

Other structural variables embedded in the program format that could have limited patient change include mundane ones such as meeting-room size and relative comfort, neither explicity reflected in the basic design of the study. Although the design of the study did not take such variables into account, they are not irrelevant to the planning of future studies of the effective volunteer. Each is a potential source of influence on outcome that can be confounded with the independent variables presumably under examination.

Given these limitations, only a few student leader characteristics were found to relate to patient change. These exceptions occurred primarily in the weak, but tantalizing relations between the GAIT "therapeutic talent" ratings (and two of its components: warmth and understanding) and improvement in ward behavior, using the average percentage of improvement method. These qualities, as judged behaviorally in group sessions with fellow students, related discriminably to patient improvement. Although the relations were far from solid, perhaps diluted by factors already discussed, they were among the few hints in the present data of volunteer attributes that may predict to positive change in chronic schizophrenics exposed to a program such as the present one.

The GAIT measures were the only "personality" indices used in the study based on *actual observed behavior* as opposed to verbal statements *about* behavior reflected in paper and pencil, or single ratings based on brief tape segments. Perhaps, *behavioral* qualities such as warmth and understanding, consensually judged by peers and trained observers, are sufficiently basic to generalize to group contacts with patients, and thus to relate to outcome indices involving improved patient behavior on the wards.

II. STUDENT LEADERS VERSUS NONVOLUNTEER CONTROLS: PERSONALITY MEASURES

The issue of concern in this section is the extent to which student leaders who volunteered for this program differed in personality make-up from nonvolunteer controls. Prior work in this area (e.g., Knapp & Holzberg, 1964) indicates that such differences, if any, are small. A basis for examining E versus C differences was available through the extensive test battery given to the 30 student leaders and 61 SC IIs drawn from introductory psychology classes. This battery yielded a total of 49 subscale scores from the PRF, Chapin, A–B, I–E, Self-disclosure, Wrightsman, and ACL measures.

First, differences between the mean scores of male and female leaders in the E group were tested for significance. Only four such differences were found (Chinsky, 1968). Females had higher scores than males on PRF sentience and nurturance, and lower scores on PRF aggression and they endorsed more adjectives on the ACL self-confidence scale. Given the total number of comparisons (49), the number of significant sex differences (4) did not exceed chance. We thus assumed that there were no systematic differences between the sex subgroups in the student-leader sample and pooled them for the major analyses.

Table 6.5 presents means and standard deviations for the total student E-group for all 49 personality-related measures. The significance of the differences between the E-group means and those of the C-group (SC II) was tested individually for all 49 variables. Only four significant differences emerged from this analysis, with Es having higher social insight scores on the Chapin, self-disclosure scores on the Jourard, A scores on the A–B scale, and PRF nurturance scores (Chinsky, 1968). Once again, the pattern of four significant differences in a series of 49 comparisons does not exceed chance. Consistent with the earlier findings of Knapp and Holzberg (1964) growing out of a similar program, we conclude that there are few personality differences between students who volunteer for human-service programs and those who do not. Certainly, there is no support in the present findings for the concern voiced by some that such programs run the risk of attracting especially upset or disturbed students. Given

TABLE 6.5 *Means and Standard Deviations for E Group on Forty-Nine Personality Measures*

	Variable	*M*	*SD*		Variable	*M*	*SD*
1.	PRF—Affiliation	15.0	3.2	25.	Self-disclosure	42.2	2.9
2.	PRF—Order	8.3	4.1	26.	Wrightsman Favorability	103.4	35.8
3.	PRF—Exhibition	11.2	3.3	27.	Wrightsman Individual difference	124.6	11.3
4.	PRF—Dependence	7.5	3.1	28.	ACL—Favorability	46.9	11.0
5.	PRF—Impulsivity	11.4	3.4	29.	ACL—Unfavorability	51.5	8.6
6.	PRF—Succorance	9.0	3.8	30.	ACL—Self-confidence	46.0	8.8
7.	PRF—Sentience	16.6	2.3	31.	ACL—Self-control	45.0	10.1
8.	PRF—Dominance	9.8	3.8	32.	ACL—Liability	53.3	12.6
9.	PRF—Play	11.6	2.4	33.	ACL—Personal adjustment	44.5	10.6
10.	PRF—Autonomy	9.0	2.9	34.	ACL—Achievement	47.0	8.8
11.	PRF—Understanding	13.6	2.6	35.	ACL—Dominance	47.0	9.8
12.	PRF—Endurance	10.8	3.9	36.	ACL—Endurance	47.1	12.1
13.	PRF—Aggression	6.9	3.5	37.	ACL—Order	48.8	11.7
14.	PRF—Change	12.3	3.0	38.	ACL—Intraception	53.6	9.6
15.	PRF—Social recognition	10.3	3.2	39.	ACL—Nurturance	47.8	10.3
16.	PRF—Abasement	6.0	2.5	40.	ACL—Affiliation	44.7	10.5
17.	PRF—Cognitive structure	9.0	3.5	41.	ACL—Heterosexuality	50.2	8.8
18.	PRF—Nurturance	14.3	3.3	42.	ACL—Exhibition	50.3	10.9
19.	PRF—Harm avoidance	8.1	4.0	43.	ACL—Autonomy	51.0	10.8
20.	PRF—Achievement	11.4	3.4	44.	ACL—Aggression	52.6	10.4
21.	PRF—Social desirability	15.0	2.6	45.	ACL—Change	50.9	12.2
22.	Chapin	27.3	3.7	46.	ACL—Succorance	51.3	9.8
23.	A-B	14.7	3.1	47.	ACL—Abasement	52.3	9.7
24.	I-E	10.0	3.3	48.	ACL—Deference	50.1	10.3
				49.	ACL—Defensiveness	45.1	9.9

the fact that the E group was slightly older, and further along in college than the Cs, the differences between them were remarkably few.

III. STUDENT LEADERS VERSUS NONVOLUNTEER CONTROLS: INITIAL ATTITUDES AND ATTITUDE CHANGE

A. Initial Attitudes

Eleven measures were used to compare initial attitudes and change in attitudes in our several student groups. Two of these were the overall "favorable" and "unfavorable" ACL scales derived from student ratings of the "typical mental hospital patient." The other nine were semantic differential measures based on ratings of the following concepts: "mental patient," "mental hospital," "myself," "average person," "nurses," "psychologists," "psychotherapy," "mental illness," and "volunteer groups" (see Table 4.6).

Subjects used in the comparison of initial group attitudes included the 30 student Es, 30 SC Is, and 30 *S*s drawn randomly from the larger group of 61 SC IIs. Presented in Table 6.6 are means and standard deviations for these three groups on the 11 attitude measures, taken before the experiment started. Cursory examination of this table indicates that the three groups were, in the main, comparable with respect to initial attitudes. A three-by-one simple analysis of variance (Winer, 1962) was computed for each variable, testing for the significance of differences among group means. While several overall significant differences emerged from the analyses on the SD concepts "average person," "mental patient," and "mental illnesss," refined analysis demonstrated that these were attributable to differences between the two control groups (Chinsky, 1968). Initial E-group attitudes were thus not systematically different either from those of SC I or SC II. Similarly, within the E group, no differences were found between males and females on any of the attitude measures. The present group of student leaders was not more idealistic than its fellows; indeed, it manifested overall attitudes highly comparable to those of student peers. This similarity of initial attitudes is consistent with the earlier findings of Turner, Holzberg, and Knapp (1967).

B. Attitude Change

Attitude measures were available for Es, SC Is and SC IIs at three points; before the program started, while it was in progress, and after it had ended. The question of prime concern in this analysis was whether differential attitude

TABLE 6.6 *Mean Values and Standard Deviations of Initial Attitudes for Volunteer Group, Control I, and Control II*[a]

Attitude concept	Volunteer group		Control I		Control II	
	M	*SD*	*M*	*SD*	*M*	*SD*
ACL—Patient favorable	16.4	9.0	16.1	9.4	16.5	8.4
ACL—Patient unfavorable	82.2	14.7	80.4	14.5	81.1	18.2
SD—Nurses	75.7	9.7	80.0	10.0	78.2	8.4
SD—Volunteer groups	77.0	7.4	74.5	8.8	75.8	10.6
SD—Mental illness	44.4	8.1	45.0	6.6	40.2	6.2
SD—Average person	64.2	10.2	71.4	5.7	66.8	9.3
SD—Psychotherapy	70.8	7.3	67.8	8.2	66.7	9.3
SD—Psychologist	75.5	8.2	75.5	7.2	71.5	8.6
SD—Myself	73.8	7.0	76.4	8.0	74.9	10.9
SD—Mental patient	46.7	7.8	52.3	5.1	43.7	8.4
SD—Mental hospital	60.8	10.5	64.6	10.2	59.8	8.5

[a] $N = 90$: 30 Volunteer; 30 Control I; 30 Control II.

change took place among the three groups as a function of Es having actively participated in the program. This question was examined using a two-way factorial analysis of variance with repeated measures (Winer, 1962). A series of significant, internally consistent findings emerged from these analyses. These data are presented, respectively, for ACL "Patient Favorability" Scale (see Table 6.7), the ACL "Patient Unfavorability" Scale (see Table 6.8) and the SD concepts of "mental patient" (see Table 6.9), and "mental hospital" (see Table 6.10). In each case, the analysis of variance summary table and the nine group-mean scores (three groups and three time periods) are presented.

For the ACL patient favorability measure (Table 6.7), the three groups had essentially identical scores at the prepoint. By the second assessment, when the program had been in progress for 1 month, Es had significantly higher patient favorability scores than both C groups, a difference that remained at the posttest point. On this measure, Es sharply verbalized more positive attitudes after the program, while both C groups held constant over time. Precisely the opposite held true for the ACL patient-unfavorability scale (Table 6.8). By the second testing period, Es showed a sharp decrease in unfavorable attitudes which continued through the postprogram evaluation point. On the SD concept "mental patient," (Table 6.9) student leaders again had the most favorable attitudes at the end of the project even though they had started from an initial base of directionally less favorable attitudes than did the two C groups (significantly so, in one case). The overall pattern of more positive attitudes for student leaders and stable attitudes for Cs was also found on this measure. Finally, student leader attitudes toward "mental hospitals" (Table 6.10) became sharply more

TABLE 6.7 *Analysis of Variance for E versus C Groups on ACL Patient-Favorability Scale*

Source	*SS*	*df*	*MS*	*F*
Between subjects				
Groups	1822.69	2	911.34	5.82**
Subjects within groups	13606.84	87	156.40	
Within subjects				
Time	644.45	2	332.22	8.04**
Groups X Time	919.59	4	229.89	5.56**
Time X Subjects within groups	7183.28	174	41.28	

Mean Scores[a]

	Groups X Time periods		
	Time 1	Time 2	Time 3
Vol. group	16.4	25.7	24.6
Control I	16.1	16.4	17.5
Control II	16.5	16.5	17.2

[a] N=30 for all groups.
** $p < .01$.

negative following program participation. There was a linear trend through assessment points two and three. Both C groups maintained stable attitudes to the concept mental hospitals. At the end, E group attitudes toward mental hospitals were distinctly less favorable than those of the two C groups.

An analysis by *scales* of the SD concepts "mental patients" and "mental hospital" allows for more specific examination of attitude change toward these two concepts. Using the same factorial design for each of the scales, it was found that Es saw mental patients as significantly more pleasant, less harmful, more predictable, more friendly, and more passive at the end of the program than did Cs. The last of these changes was directionally opposed to their overall favorable change in attitude toward the mental patient. The E group saw the "mental hospital" as significantly more passive, more cold, less helpful, less good, less pleasant, less interesting, less friendly, and less effective than did Cs, at the end of the program.

On all remaining concepts, differences among groups in attitude change over time failed to reach statistical significance. For example, SD attitudes toward "myself," "psychologists," "nurses," and "volunteer groups" did not change differentially across groups. Initially, high positive student-attitudes on all of those measures limited the possibility of such change. For any SD scale,

TABLE 6.8 *Analysis of Variance for E versus C Groups on ACL Patient-Unfavorability Scale*

Source	*SS*	*df*	*MS*	*F*
Between subjects				
Groups	3151.31	2	1575.65	2.58
Subjects within groups	53126.88	87	610.65	
Within subjects				
Time	2194.49	2	1097.24	11.70**
Groups X Time	2878.85	4	719.71	7.67**
Time X Subjects within groups	16307.30	174	93.72	

Mean Scores[a]

	Groups X Time periods		
	Time 1	Time 2	Time 3
Vol. group	82.2	65.8	69.3
Control I	80.4	82.7	77.5
Control II	81.1	78.8	77.2

[a] $N = 30$ for all groups.
** $p < .01$.

the maximum theoretical score was 98, and some average initial group scores exceeded 75 (see Table 6.6). Thus, there was relatively little room for further positive change.

The absence of significant change differences between E and C on the remaining attitude measures serves as an incidental control. It reduces the likelihood that the significant observed changes might be due to the E groups general tendency to have responded in a socially desirable manner to all concepts (Rundquist, 1966; Edwards, 1959). Thus, for example, while student leaders' overall attitudes toward "mental patients" improved sharply, their attitudes toward "mental illness" stayed constant. The sense of this argument is that the positive changes in leader attitudes following program participation, were genuine in the central areas in which they took place. They cannot readily be discounted as a function of methodological artifact or extraneous variables. Indeed, E leaders were able to evaluate separately the mental hospital per se, patients, and the hospital staff.

Conclusions about differential attitude change in student leaders cluster around two major areas. First, as a result of participating in the program, students developed more positive attitudes to patients. This finding accords well

TABLE 6.9 *Analysis of Variance for E versus C Groups on SD Mental Patient Concept*

Source	*SS*	*df*	*MS*	*F*
Between subjects				
Groups	2446.58	2	1223.29	11.26**
Subjects within groups	9452.41	87	108.64	
Within Subjects				
Time	218.69	2	109.34	3.45*
Groups X Time	641.21	4	160.30	5.06**
Time X Subjects within groups	5506.74	174	31.64	

Mean scores[a]

	Group X Time periods		
	Time 1	Time 2	Time 3
Vol. group	46.7	51.3	53.6
Control I	52.3	51.3	50.8
Control II	43.7	44.5	45.0

[a]$N = 30$ for all groups.
*$p < .05$. **$p < .01$.

with the earlier data of Scheibe (1965) and Turner *et al* (1967). Contact seems to have reduced threat, and, after considerable interaction with patients, students see them more favorably and in less stereotypic, socially undesirable ways. Student leaders also developed less favorable attitudes toward the institution of the mental hopsital following their program experience. This finding closely resembles one reported earlier by Cowen, Zax, and Laird (1966), whose student volunteers evaluated the concept "elementary schools" more negatively after having participated in an after-school companionship program for primary graders with school adjustment problems. Students in human service programs seem to identify, easily and strongly with those whom they serve—whether mental hospital patients or young school children. As they see these target individuals in close contact and come to understand their circumstances better, a force is set into motion by which some portion of the person's adverse condition is attributed to the setting in which he is being seen. It is certainly not difficult to build such connections in the traditional mental hospital. What ensues, is an attribution of blame for the individual's circumstances to the institution and, with it, a directionally negative change in attitude to that setting.

TABLE 6.10 *Analysis of Variance for E versus C Groups on SD Mental Hospital Concept*

Source	*SS*	*df*	*MS*	*F*
Between subjects				
Groups	4912.05	2	2456.03	13.63**
Subjects within groups	15670.09	87	180.11	
Within subjects				
Time	2433.69	2	1216.84	24.16**
Groups X Time	1817.30	4	454.32	9.02**
Time X Subjects within groups	8761.66	174	50.35	

Mean Scores[a]

	Groups X Time periods		
	Time 1	Time 2	Time 3
Vol. group	60.8	50.6	44.8
Control I	64.6	61.6	60.8
Control II	59.8	59.0	58.0

[a]N = 30 for all groups.
**$p < .01$.

Finally, we note that where significant attitude change took place in student leaders, such change was in evidence early in the program and remained stable over time. Early contact experiences are apparently the most influential ones, at least insofar as the attitudes tapped in the present study are concerned.

IV. GROUP PROCESS MEASURES

A. Changes in Group Process over Time

An overall description of how patient groups spent their time, derived from the GAF, was presented in Table 5.2. Another question to be raised is the extent to which this group profile changed over the course of the program. Table 5.2 also gives mean percentages of time spent by groups in each of the nine activity categories for the first, second, and third parts of the program. These data are remarkably stable. No single activity category changed in frequency by more than 4% from any one time period to any other. In part, this stability reflects the lack of mobility and limitations of equipment and supplies which sharply restricted what the groups could do. Whatever the reason, there was virtually no change in activity patterns across time periods. Therefore, the "total" process figures are used in further substantive analyses, since they accurately reflect time-allocations for all periods of the overall sequence.

There is another general way to assess change in process over time. When volunteers submitted GAF forms, they also rated overall group behavior on a five-point rating scale ranging from "rarely good" (point 1) to "almost always good" (point 5) (see Table 4.3). Changes in these overall process judgments across the three time-periods were tested using a three by one simple analysis of variance (Winer, 1962). The results of this analysis (Chinsky, 1968) indicate that student leaders judged significant improvement in group behavior ($F = 13.51$, $p = .01$) during the program. The mean initial group rating was 3.56, whereas the mean final group rating was 4.40. These objective findings are buttressed by observations made by student leaders in the diary-accounts of their program experiences (to be discussed in Chapter 7). These statements revealed more positive feelings by students toward their groups as the program developed, stronger group identification and sense of cohesiveness, as well as easier conversation and an increase in interpersonal interactions. The following is an illustrative statement made by one volunteer to justify his higher rating of the group processes in the later stages of the program: "The patients trust me more and are more enthusiastic. [There is]. . .greater group unity and participation in activities. Conversation is much easier. Most of the women feel more comfortable among themselves and will often question each other freely."

Findings reported in the above section suggest that although the mean percentage of time spent in various activities did not change during the course of the program, the quality of relationships among group members and between patients and group leaders improved.

B. Volunteer Attributes and Process Measures

Scores for the 30 student leaders on the Truax-Carkhuff measures, the A-B, the combined GAIT ratings, and the six derived factors were correlated with the average time spent by their groups in each of the nine GAF categories. These correlations using student attributes as predictors, and process indices as criteria are summarized elsewhere (Chinsky, 1968). Student attributes did not relate systematically to *any* group activity. Conceivably, factors such as particular group needs, physical constraints, and limiting hospital regulations reduced the potential for finding such relationships. These factors have been cited in the section dealing with observed high-stability of process categories over the program time subperiods.

Group activities were determined not solely by the volunteer, but also by patient needs and desires. Physical activities, for example, occurred more frequently in male groups, whereas preparing food was, understandably, more common in female groups. Beyond the influence of group preferences or needs, certain activities (e.g., physical ones) were limited for all groups, by confined meeting quarters. Other activities (e.g., table games) probably occured *more* frequently for the same reason—i.e., they were among the few that could be comfortably managed under the circumstances—a reality constraint unrelated to volunteer personality attributes. Restrictions such as little freedom on the hospital grounds and the inability to leave the grounds further curtailed the range of activities available to groups.

C. Process Measures and Outcome

In order to determine whether what groups actually did related to patient change, the amount of time spent by patient groups in each of the nine process categories was correlated both with performance and ward-behavior change scores. With 10 performance change measures plus an overall performance change estimate, the first of these matrices was 9 X 11, and with five ward behavior changes scores, the second was a 9 X 5 matrix.

Although the overall number of significant correlations between process categories and ward improvement scores did not exceed chance (Chinsky, 1968), 12 of the 99 correlations between process activities and performance improvement scores were significant (see Table 6.11). This number *does* exceed chance expectancy; moreover, the pattern of significant correlations was internally consistent and informative. For example, time spent by groups *talking* related to improvement on two measures of perceptual functioning. The converse of this was even clearer. Time spent by groups *listening* (defined as "times when the group is passive, listening to a record, a poem you are reading, an instrument, etc.") related negatively to patient improvement on several perceptual, psychomotor, and perceptual-motor indices as well as to the overall patient performance improvement index.

The relations found between specific group activities and patient improvement indices suggest several explanations. The first comes from an observation without supporting objective data, that talking occurred most often in groups with rapport both among patients and between patients and student leaders. Talking, especially involving a person from the outside world, may be a substantial and pleasant departure from the characteristically dull hospital routine (see pages 24 and 155).

Listening, typically to TV and radio, on the other hand is far from an atypical experience for patients; it is very much part of their repetitive day-to-day routine. A relatively high listening rate in a group may have reflected poor patient–patient and student–patient rapport. Such passive activity precludes genuine group participation. It is reasonable to suppose that active engagement

TABLE 6.11 *Correlation of Process Measures with Group Mean Improvement Scores: Performance Measures*

	Process measures								
Outcome measures	Eating	Talking	Music	Listening	Artistic activities	Table games	Physical activities	Individual activities	Quiet times
RT 1	.15	.19	.24	.06	−.25	−.21	.07	.40*	.19
RT 2	.00	−.02	−.26	−.07	−.25	.07	.38*	.17	−.01
TAPS	−.28	.32	.10	−.67**	−.05	−.16	−.44*	.07	.00
Digit symbol	−.19	.24	−.09	−.36*	.13	.12	−.24	−.18	−.06
Verbal fluency	−.40*	−.12	−.09	−.08	−.10	.45*	.19	−.17	.00
Stroop A	−.10	.24	−.16	−.39*	−.03	−.09	−.11	−.22	.15
Stroop B	−.16	.23	.11	−.33	.11	−.21	−.13	−.29	.09
Stroop C	−.14	.44*	−.23	−.22	.00	−.24	.02	−.06	−.08
Stroop total	−.22	.41*	−.01	−.22	.05	−.29	−.07	−.22	.19
Figure ground	−.05	−.09	.14	−.15	.36*	−.10	−.05	.00	.20
Performance total	−.27	.32	−.05	−.52**	−.11	.02	−.06	−.09	.12

$^{*}p < .05$. $^{**}p < .01$.

›f the environment, as opposed to sitting back passively facilities the type of "waking-up" effect reflected in patient improvement on several performance measures. Thus, there is some evidence to suggest that what students and patients actually *do* together has potential impact for patient change.

Chapter 7

THE PROJECT FROM A HUMAN PERSPECTIVE

I. INTRODUCTION

Every research project, whether based on laboratory or clinical intervention, is marked by incidents and human problems that do not reach the pages of professional journals and books. Beginning researchers are often surprised to learn that, like most jobs, scientific investigation is filled with ups and downs, mistakes and joys that are rarely reported in the "methods section." It is these informal learning experiences that prompt faculty members to tell their students that the only real way to learn about research is to do it. This is especially true in clinical investigations. Many important hypothesis-finding (as opposed to hypothesis-testing), "breakthroughs" come from experience gained in implementing and conducting a project. Much of the "meat" of a service project lies in everyday human encounters that are integral to "relevant" research and yet extremely difficult to communicate scientifically.

Having completed the "scientific" description of our project, this chapter will attempt to convey the experiential aspect of our work. This approach may help prospective mental health volunteers, college students and others, to sense a portion of the total experience that may be especially meaningful to them. For volunteers about to undertake human-service activities, especially in institutional settings, this chapter may serve as a vicarious journey. It is the sort of "coming attractions" that many of our own students would have welcomed prior to their experience. To volunteer workers who have already participated in human-service activities, perhaps this account will add a measure of perspective. For professional colleagues either involved in, or considering similar projects, the chapter is offered as a description of "real life" encounters we faced–from the entirely enjoyable to the utterly vexing. Hopefully, reflecting on such experiences will help better to understand the past and to plan for the future.

In sum, the purpose of this chapter is to describe the program from an informal standpoint–an account of project evolution and processes as they personally affected the authors, students, patients, and hospital staff. To do this, we shall use clinical observations, tape recordings from group sessions, student diaries, anecdotal incidents, and other impressionistic data. Wherever possible, original student notes will be quoted verbatim, in order to preserve the actual flavor of the experience. Although some of the material to be presented in this chapter may have appeared elsewhere in the volume, we wish here to convey an overview of the project from the human perspective. The preliminary stages of our investigations–the pilot study, formal course arrangements, and administrative hurdles–were described in detail in Chapter 2. The present narrative begins with the initial phase of the main study.

II. THE "TUNE-UP" PERIOD

Following the selection of 48 students for the school and state hospital programs, there was a 10-week process of preparation for "the encounters," based both on formal and informal class meetings–lectures and discussion. The authors, and an advanced graduate student, presented a theoretical rationale for use of nonprofessionals and considered other current mental health issues and problems reflected in the reading materials described in Table 2.1. While some students enjoyed the classroom orientation and most tolerated it, neither a feeling of personal involvement nor a sense of clinical responsibility was established as a result of orientation.

A. "Sensitizing"

The GAIT sessions, which took place during the final phases of the 10-week course (see page 31 for a detailed description of GAIT) had a fortuitous, but nevertheless important, positive impact in the "tuning-up" process. This approach had a powerful "sensitizing" effect both on student participants and staff. At the end of each 90–120-minute session, almost every group member was highly gratified by the experience. Most expressed strong feelings of having been personally moved by the sessions. A sense of friendship, beyond that common to classmates, was much in evidence, as were expressions of comradeship and feelings of purpose and mission. At the end of each session, the authors asked the students how they had felt revealing personal problems to teachers and supervisors. The feelings of many are well conveyed in the half-serious, half-facetious introspection of one student, which illuminates the nature of the unfolding supervisor–supervisee relationship. "You revealed yourselves in front of the class, so why should we feel hesitant to reveal ourselves here?"

Just before patient contact began we invited the two female students who had been the summer pilot-group leaders to talk to the other students about their experiences. They, together with a first-year graduate student who had served as an undergraduate companion in the Connecticut Valley State Hospital Project (Holzberg *et al.*, 1967), were doubtless more effective in alleviating concerns about "impending doom" than the authors had been. Their perceptions and insights were of considerable help to students anxiously anticipating the clinical experience. In retrospect, the use of "veteran volunteers" as consultants to new recruits makes good sense both clinically and administratively.

III. INITIATION DAY

The final act in preparing for patient contact was a group tour of hospital facilities. The focus of the program was in three of the four hospital buildings housing chronic patients. Failure to include the fourth building was due to the program's having been deftly "locked out" by professionals on that unit. At that time, this rebuff was perceived by the authors as a gross failure. Only after the program was over and we were able to think back rationally, did we develop a more measured view of what had taken place (see Chapter 2, page 46).

Our tour of the project buildings took place on a dreary November day. The students had heard about the hospital from the Chief of the Psychology Department and the supervisor of hospital volunteers, who had informed them, in general terms, about hospital routine and regulations. The authors had also given the students some idea of what to expect. Nevertheless, most students had never seen a mental hospital before and only a very few had been inside Rochester State (despite the fact that it was only 1.5 miles from campus). All volunteers met on campus and drove to the hospital together. We congregated in the relatively new, acute-treatment building, where arrangements for the tour were made. The students were divided into small groups to visit the specific buildings and wards in which they would be working. As we approached Building O (see Figure 7.1), a stark, gray, unimpressive structure, the mood of the volunteers paralleled the weather. (In fact, Building O had the best physical features of the three.) The other two buildings, H1 and H2, were large, brownstone, two-story structures, connected with a long ground-level corridor. Building H1 had eight wards, each with 60–70 female patients. Building H2 housed about 300 males and four of its wards were occupied by "severely disturbed female" patients. In contrast to the "new" building we had just left, these were truly "back-wards."

As the students proceeded on the tour, the authors could not help but notice a cloud of silence and depression, not unlike our own feelings when we first encountered the dank chronic wards of the state hospital. Although by now reasonably well-accustomed to the hospital's stark environment, the authors could nevertheless readily recall, with considerable ill-ease, the earlier experience searching for patients identified in the files, for pretest evaluation. On more than one occasion during these searches, patients were literally lifted from the bathroom floor, where the overworked attendant had left them in order to cope with a disturbance created at the opposite end of the ward. Nevertheless, at some point in the "professional socialization process" we had learned to dim our responses to the impoverished human condition of chronic hospitalized patients.

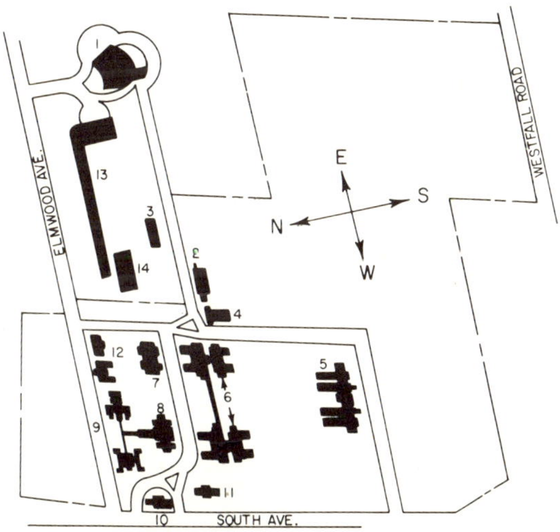

Figure 7.1. Rochester State Hospital. Key: 1. Medical and acute treatment building; 2. Powerhouse; 3. Storehouse; 4. Laundry; 5. Building O; 6. Building H1, Building H2; 7. Auditorium; 8. Livingston building; 9. Reception and Building D; 10. Administration; 11. Physician's home; 12. Nurses home; 13. Rehabilitation center; 14. Chapel of St. Jude.

Fortunately, our student volunteers had not learned to suppress this entirely human reaction.

Overcrowded dormitories, with beds so closely arranged that privacy was impossible, were among the first things noticed by the students. Worn, resigned faces of long-term patients passively regarded the students. Occasionally a patient approached one of the students with the result that everyone felt self-conscious. This "visit-to-the-zoo" feeling made us wish we had decided against a tour. Yet had we not done this before the program started, the same shock, disbelief, and revulsion would merely have become part of the initial session. At least the tour provided a bit of time for students to harden themselves for the initial session.

Despite overcrowded conditions, socialization on the wards was minimal. The absence of interpersonal interaction was due in part to the custodial orientation of the hospital and in part to the heavy use of drugs. The custodial orientation was abetted by the physical arrangement of a single large room lined with chairs to the wall. More important, there did not seem to be any reason for interaction and most patients simply did not have the social skills needed to interact with others. With the exception of other volunteer groups (e.g., the "gray ladies") who provided "social hours," very little took place on the wards, save the inevitable droning of the television set—sometimes in little more than a *pro forma* way. This first glimpse of hospital life, while both frightening and depressing for many students, also served as a powerful catalyst for enthusiasm and active seeking of possibilities for providing a significant addition to the empty lives of the patients.

Among the early questions the students asked us was: "What do the patients do?" The ward routine was typical: Up at 7:00; breakfast and medication; sit or help to clean the ward; lunch at 11:30; sit; dinner at 5:00; sit; and to bed between 7:30 and 9:00. The students came to see their role quite accurately, as initiators of human interaction. Over the course of the year, as patient interaction increased, the initial pessimism of the students yielded, first to euphoria at any, even minor hint of success and eventually, to a more realistic appraisal of their impact and limitations.

IV. FINDING THE MEETING ROOMS

The program format required fairly sizable rooms where patient–student groups could meet. At least seven rooms were needed and, given the overcrowded conditions of the hospital, there was no overabundance of these. The basement of H2 afforded the only possibility in either H1 or H2. This meant that the H1 patients had to be brought down the long tunnel-like connecting corridor to the H2 basement rooms.This nightly march was reminiscent of an old prisoner-of-war movie. The scene was one of old clothes, worn faces mirroring depression and apathy, dragging feet echoing down a dark tunnel, the rancid odors of institutional food from the nearby kitchens, and food left on the plates of women already too heavy from their excessively starchy diet. Indeed, to us one striking measure of program success was the perceptible change in this marching scene over time. By mid-year, there were more smiling, laughing faces. Better grooming was evident. Feet lifted a little higher and rather than marching single-file, patients walked together in small groups. En route, they seemed to anticipate, with some happiness, the interactions of their group meetings. There was *something* for them to look forward to.

Five appropriately sized rooms were found in the H2 basement. One had been used as a library and storage room. A second, unoccupied at night, was the recreational therapy department's game room; it contained some recreational supplies. A third room, used during the day as an employee's lounge and dining area, had a sink and a refrigerator. The fourth was a small sitting room. The fifth room had not been used at all, and was, with its gray cement floor and walls, the most barren of all. Two additional rooms were found in Building O. One, used as a daytime employee meeting room, was about as large as a wide bowling alley. The other was a small lounge.

One of the first tasks that the students set for themselves was to brighten up the physical surroundings in what came to be thought of as "their" rooms. Together with "their" patients they covered the walls with pictures, brought in surplus furniture, including a rug! Thus, it was, with an odd mixture of depression, and a sense of purpose and enthusiasm, that the project was launched.

V. SCHEDULING THE MEETINGS

However mundane, one of the more difficult administrative problems was to decide when the groups should meet. Some patients performed hospital duties during the day, usually as kitchen-aides or in the laundry. A handful either worked off the grounds or had city privileges. The meeting rooms were occupied at various, unpredictable, daytime hours. Thus, daytime groups were particularly difficult to schedule.

Since patients had to be up for breakfast at 7:00 a.m., and since frequently there was only one attendant for as many as 60–70 patients, it was both necessary and efficient, in the custodial sense, to have the patients asleep as early as possible. In the evenings, most patients were in bed before 9:00 p.m. Indeed, before the program started, some wards turned off their lights at 7:30 p.m. Thus, late evening meetings were impossible.

For practical reasons, then, we decided that the groups should meet in the early evenings between 6:00 and 8:30 p.m. This was a time of day when patients uniformly had nothing to do. These hours were also most convenient for hospital staff and students. It was the time when regular routine would be least "disrupted," a source of great concern to the staff.

As reported in Chapter 2, we were also able to persuade hospital administration to hire overtime personnel for these early evening hours to escort the patients to their meeting rooms. During the day it would have been impossible to find additional staff. Furthermore, the meeting rooms were free during the evenings. Once we were able to convince the ward staff not to turn the lights off at 7:30, our groups had finally found a place in the state hospital "routine"—the period between 6:00 and 8:30 p.m., Monday through Thursday. This was a major accomplishment. From the students' standpoint, these hours did not conflict with class times, and consequently no special arrangements were needed because of schedule conflicts.

Since some groups met from 6:00 to 7:00 p.m., and others from 7:20 to 8:20, on occasion some of the "second shift" students arrived early. In the evenings, the H2 building was in the charge of an elderly nursing supervisor. One student made it a habit to drop by early to see her. The woman was a widow who lived alone with her cat, an animal that had reached the unbelievable age of 20. She and the student frequently "small-talked" about cats, which she admired unstintingly. Every day after dinner, supervisor and student helped a very old female patient, not a project participant, gather leftover meat which they, together, put on the front lawn for the stray cats who were regular visitors. After a time, the student began to bring his own cat to the group meetings, always being sure to stop by to let the supervisor greet it properly. The patients enjoyed the animal and came to regard it as a "member" of their group. While this may have been a perfectly fine idea, the authors did not learn how it began until much later in the year. One night the supervisor told one of us that her ancient pet cat had died, and since then, a student had brought in his cat for her. She tearfully related how her own cat, acquired before her husband's death, had reminded her of him, how lonely she had been since its death, and how much she appreciated the student bringing his pet to the hospital. Thus, though intended for the benefit of patients, it was clear that the program had utility in unexpected quarters.

Twenty-eight groups met in the early evening, twice weekly, and four others met during the day. The latter were scheduled during several free, odd hours on Tuesday and Thursday afternoons. Thus, a total of 64 group meetings were arranged each week. The daytime groups were led by four coeds who were not free evenings. These four developed their own self-contained sense of identity. They traveled to the hospital together and became well known to the daytime staff. They were eventually so much considered a part of the staff they were permitted to have their own keys and to gather their own groups together from the various wards. To be given keys in a state hospital is tantamount to being given an honorary degree from a university or a key to a city from the mayor.

VI. STUDENT REACTIONS

From the beginning of the program, each student was asked to keep a "diary" of ongoing impressions. Students were encouraged to be as open about their feelings as possible. These diaries, which included initial impressions, descriptions of group sessions throughout the program, and notes pertaining to termination, were collected at the end of the year.

Although reactions of students to the first hospital visit, as indicated in discussion meetings and diary notes, were varied, some general features can be noted. Many were disillusioned and depressed even though they had been prepared intellectually for the experience. Others, though they found the situation to be unfortunate, had more or less expected this to be the case. Several typical student reactions to the initial visits, as excerpted verbatim from diaries, are presented below:

PETER: *Inspection day—very depressing! These people look as if they have been used up and thrown away. Human trash! I felt as if I was some sort of monster when I looked into the wards. As I stood there, I could see 70 absolutely blank faces turn in my direction.*

KATY: *Well, here it is at last. First there was . . . [the new building] huge, clean, antispetic . . .. Then the tour . . .. It looked big and gray on the outside. The bars [on O building] didn't seem too reassuring. H building—antiseptic green, bare, depressing. All those old ladies just sitting around, nobody doing anything. Too many people just sitting. Outside we see men walk by on the way back to their residence. It's cold and they're poorly dressed; one doesn't have even a shirt under his ragged coat. They walk by without speaking, with heads down—maybe I should say shuffle. Pessimism.*

PENNY: *The car ride over was funny—everyone was excited and nervous, so that we joked about what we would see. After coming back to campus the car was quiet. Quite a few of us were depressed. The patients were much different than expected. Not malicious at all, but friendly and looked as though all they needed is a little (a lot!) of love. Talked to the cutest little lady—could have been someone's grandmother—probably is! That's depressing too.*

Many students were struck by the sterility of the surroundings and the locked doors.

ELAINE: *The most disturbing thing was the fact that every door had to be unlocked and relocked behind us. I can't imagine locking adults, even children, into a room, but I suppose they're [the patients] used to it.*

DONALD: *The most striking things to me were the fetish on keys that goes on, though I suppose it is necessary . . . and the fact that everyone seems to age quickly in a mental hospital. I get the impression that as one enters as a patient, one ages five years and gains a year per week till he looks and feels as old as everyone else.*

HANK: *It didn't seem possible for anyone to improve in surroundings such as this. Most of the patients were dressed fairly shabby and were doing nothing but sitting in chairs when we saw them. I felt a little apprehensive. I assume the patients "feel" the fact that they are locked in, for I too felt restrained as soon as the door was locked behind me. The building had a certain indescribable hospital smell about it. For one who had no previous exposure to a state mental hospital, I was disconcerted even though I had prepared myself for the visit.*

After having visited the hospital and having met some of the people with whom they would work, it is not surprising that the thoughts of many students shifted anxiously to the task ahead. Their reactions ranged across a wide spectrum from strong apprehension to renewed confidence of success. The majority of the impressions, however, reflected a great deal of concern. Some of the student's comments:

MARY: *It is not surprising that I find myself quite anxious about the whole situation. I am especially concerned about how I can handle a one to eight relationship. Although these people are supposed to be sick, they are still people, with eight distinct personalities.*

DONALD: *I came away a bit depressed and apprehensive about the coming weeks, but a bit more convinced that we will be enthusiastically received if for no other reason than as a change of routine and more likely as a new face and a new experience for the patients.*

ROBERT: *My first impressions of the hospital were what I was told to expect. The age of the buildings, the bars on the windows and what they symbolize succeeded in creating a morbid atmosphere. I expected to walk in and see a scene out of "The Snake Pit." The worst of it was while we waited for our "tour." A large group of men was walking from one building to another. It seemed as if they weren't even conscious of their movements, their surroundings or what their goal was. Almost no one looked up—all watched their feet move, and that was it. One was young and had a strange look in his eyes (he was the only one I saw look up) and I couldn't help think that he might evolve into what the other men around him appeared to be. The women inside were quiet, peaceful in a funny way, and friendly. But it seemed as if they were like this because there was no other way to be. I almost would rather see someone argue or do something destructive. At least it would indicate a genuine feeling. . . . I really hope the project isn't going to be adult-sitting. It seems to me that they can play cards and bingo without my presence and I'd like to be able to accomplish something, even if it's just a meaningful conversation. Of course, my impressions are based on a few minutes and therefore superficial but these people seemed so engrossed into an institutional, superficial life, that I wonder if the sincere feelings that they've had haven't been numbed to the point where they've died in the process.*

VII. THE HOSPITAL STAFF

A section of Chapter 2 considered the reactions of Rochester State personnel to getting the project started. This section will describe, in detail, individual and personal reactions of specific hospital staff members and the impact of these reactions on the program. Response to the project varied both within and across positions in the hospital status-hierarchy. Beyond the simple passive or active approval of the building supervisor, which permitted the project to come into existence, it was the ward attendant who had the power to facilitate or sabotage its objectives. Among the three building supervisors, one gave the program fairly active support, another met the program with a form of passive resistance, and the third really did not care if the program existed or not. Attendant's reactions consisted of equal parts distrust and apathy. When we first presented our ideas, the program was most commonly seen as another outside intrusion on an already overworked staff. However, given the success of the summer pilot study, we were able to find some allies on staff, who later volunteered to work overtime for the project.

Consistent with general hospital policy the role of the attendant in the program was primarily custodial. This was unfortunate, since, as a result, the program did not utilize an important potential resource that might have promoted patient improvement on the ward. However, at the outset, any attempt to have used the ward staff in other ways would at best have been difficult. Recognition of the potential value of involving ward personnel in the program led to a second project (Mace, 1969) in which attendants participated meaningfully both in program planning and in the conduct of patient group meetings. Such roles were found to be more effective in bringing about positive patient change than was continuation of a simple custodial role for the attendants. Ellsworth's (1968) recent report confirms this impression.

Even given the overall limited role of ward attendants, it is interesting to contrast staff members who volunteered for the project to those who were assigned to it, although both were paid. Volunteering or not volunteering was related, in a complex way, to the reactions of building supervisors. There was "between building variance" so that cooperative supervisors generally had cooperative ward-attendant staff. This rule was not 100% accurate and an array of human personality and attitude variables remained in evidence as a determinant of whether a given attendant did or did not volunteer for the project.

The only project-related jobs of the attendant were to bring patients to and from meetings and to be available in case they were needed during a meeting. Attendants who volunteered to participate in the project were more successful in bringing patients to the meetings than were those who did not. They were consistently more willing to talk with us while waiting around the meeting area, and wanted to learn more about the project. They went out of their way to let us know ahead of time if they could not work on a given night and, when present, they tried to become a part of the project. The attendants who did not volunteer typically regimented patients more, e.g., marching them through corridors. One even remarked proudly to the authors about how well he could "keep them in line." Volunteer aides, on the other hand, caught more of the human-interaction flavor of the meetings and their patients were returned to the ward in "happier disarray."

The importance of the summer pilot program and the work of the Chief Psychologist in bringing about a closer relation between staff and program, was discussed in Chapter 2 (see page 45). Here, it should be noted that without such a pilot venture we would not have found staff members who later became program "allies." However, despite the breakthrough inherent in the very fact that it was instituted, the program was never completely accepted by the staff, and it remained in a marginal position throughout most of its existence. Only when its end was imminent did the staff begin to ask for active continuation of the project.

VIII. THE PATIENTS

In terms of formal research appraisals, patients' reactions to students were described in some detail in Chapters 4 and 5. Clinical observations of patients during the course of the program are consistent with these findings. At the outset, patients had little idea what it would be like to relate to a college student, nor did they particularly care. While many of them thought that students would be both "fun to be with" and "like themselves," little patient enthusiasm was verbalized about the initiation of the project. Then again, the patients expressed even less enthusiasm about anything else. Occasionally one could observe a reawakened fantasy of youth spent, in a patient, but this was rare indeed. If there was any evident effect on the patients starting the program, it was anticipated anxiety over prospective social interaction.

Within the first month of the project, patient attitudes changed overtly. Those patients who dropped out of the program did so after very few sessions. A number who remained seemed to "catch fire." They became convinced that the students were really going to come to the hospital regularly rather than being casual passers-through. Although patients were informed at the outset that the program would terminate at the end of the academic year, that time seemed ages away. Many patients soon began to "wake-up." They waited eagerly in front of the locked door of the ward to go to the group meeting. They now knew the authors who visited the wards frequently and many approached them to talk about almost anything. Those not yet brave enough to dare verbal interaction, smiled from across the room. While doubtless an artifact of our own involvement, we began to "see" how much better "our" patients were than the nonparticipants.

As indicated in Chapter 5, at the end of the project, many patients saw college students as nurturant, reliable, and supportive friends—as people who genuinely cared for them. The students became truly "significant others" in the lives of patients who had been bereft of noteworthy human interaction for an average of 13 years. Whatever the harder research evaluations were to yield, the genuineness and meaningfulness of this qualitative change, in such basic human terms, seemed sufficient to justify the project.

IX. THE FIRST MEETING

By the first week in November, all the necessary groundwork had been laid for the initial student–patient meetings. This was a particularly critical moment for the program. The considerable investment in time and effort to date would have been for naught if major difficulties or insurmountable problems were encountered during these early meetings. Although data from other student-companion programs and our own work in the summer pilot study offered some general reassurance, the authors still could not accurately gauge the specific impact of such a drastically different, large-scale program on patients, students, or staff of Rochester State Hospital. Each of 32 quite naive college students was about to meet and interact with eight chronic patients, alone in a room—an unprecedented event in this particular setting. Everyone was nervous! As has been the practice in prior programs of this type, initial instructions to the students were purposefully minimal. Students were simply encouraged to "foster group interaction." They were asked not to assume artificial roles and were urged to be themselves and to "act naturally, as you would with a group of friends."

In order to satisfy building supervisors, certain "safety" precautions had to be taken. For example, at least one aide was assigned to the hall outside of the meeting rooms in case of "trouble," or to escort patients to the bathroom; however, aides were specifically told not to enter a meeting room unless asked to do so by a student. The students were truly left to rely on their own strengths and resources. Throughout, the authors had sought to instill a sense of confidence in them and to reassure them that they could handle the group meetings effectively. We hoped that we had communicated this sense of confidence. Despite their understandable situational anxiety, we hoped that, at least in part, they felt some assurance. From prior discussions, both formal and informal, we had reason to believe that the students were ready, but the true test of their mettle remained to take place in actual "front-line" service.

Other potential problems lay just below the surface. Would the patients be ready for the program? Would they be willing to come to the meeting rooms? Problems of a more practical nature were also considered: Would it be possible to run so many groups simultaneously? How much time would be needed to assemble a group of patients in a meeting room? We decided to start the program slowly. Group meetings were initially held only once a week. Only female groups met the first week, followed by male groups during the second.

Then the groups began. For the most part, the vast array of potential and fantasied problems did not materialize. Physical problems were minimal. As noted in Chapter 2, in the first few weeks, the patients were convened by the authors. In general, they were ready for the group meetings and many came willingly to them. Some patients, however, were found sleeping on the wards and others were not there at all. Several night-attendants claimed that they had no knowledge of any program for which patients were supposed to be ready. This was probably true in some cases, notwithstanding repeated announcements about the program. Messages in a state hospital have an uncanny way of being lost or forgotten. Other attendants were probably too busy to pay attention to the notice. Still others did not want to be bothered. The extent of the attendant's cooperation was, as suggested earlier, often related to the reaction of his particular building supervisor.

Some patients resisted coming to the meetings. If the attendant had not previously mentioned anything to them, their initial information about the groups came the night of the first meeting. In fact, virtually all patients had been informed of the project following pretesting, but many had forgotten. There was little control over how the program was introduced to the patients by ward staff. Many had no idea of what to expect. Some were frightened.

After the purpose of the meetings had been explained to patients and after they had been told that some valued reward (e.g., free cigarettes, cake, friendly companionship, etc.) was available, the majority did go to the first meeting. Some, however, adamantly refused to attend, and their wishes were respected. No patient was ever forced to attend a group meeting. As reported in Chapter 5, about two-thirds of the initially identified group attended regularly. While on-the-ward "sorting" of attenders and nonattenders was handled without difficulty, during the first few weeks the scene in the basement halls of H2 often resembled a cross between Grand Central Station and the Chicago Stockyards.

Excerpts from diaries describe student reactions to the first meetings. Most reflect a great deal of anxiety on the students' part, despite prior intellectual preparation for the experience. However, some students, who had been prepared for the worst, were relieved to find that the patients were a lot more "normal" than they had believed. As documented in Chapter 6 (see page 128), student leaders shared the same initial stereotypes and expectations of mental patients as did their college peers. Actually meeting patients for the first time had a profound effect on their attitudes. Students were soon able to separate a negative reaction to the state hospital per se from their personal feelings about the patients and the staff. While the staff was seen much as anticipated, over time students attitudes toward patients became increasingly favorable, while their attitudes toward the hospital as an entity became less favorable.

The following diary selections are representative of student impressions about their first patient contacts.

NATE: *I began the evening rather frightened. The first woman to enter the room was the worst. I tried to sit and talk with her but got nothing but a strange grin. I was quite relieved when the next came in. Actually I was quite taken aback by the apparent sanity of most of the women.*

This evening we all made paper flowers. It seemed to go over pretty well; all of the women participated and one actually helped me by showing another woman how to work.

My first impression of the women hardly matched a preconceived notion I had developed. Except for the first woman I met . . . all seemed quite normal, some rather friendly!

MARLENE: *I was naturally full of curiosity at the first session—how responsive would the people be, how aware of what was going on, how favorable to my presence? I began by handing out decorated slips of paper to be used as name tags, and everyone except Paul filled them out and pinned them on their shirts. For about half an hour I asked them where they came from, and what kind of work they were doing before they came to Rochester State. They seemed fairly friendly and amenable, much to my surprise, and I ended the hour with a paper-and-pencil game of fold-down pictures, passed from left to right, in which each drew a head, then folded down the paper, passed it on, drew a neck and arms, etc. They were rather amused, perhaps partly for my sake.*

The students realized they had to deal with each patient as an individual as well as dealing with patients as a group. They also quickly became aware of the difficulties in this process.

PATRICIA: *When I first walked into the reading room, I asked the group to sit down and I introduced myself. I was constantly conscious of not playing favorites and tried to talk to all of them. I think my mistake was trying to treat them as a group. These men were isolated people . . . I tried to bring the group together too quickly which is something that will take a very long time and then may only be partially successful.*

One of the students noted aspects of the complex interaction between herself and her patients at the very first session. Many patients did not want to appear "different" or "sick" to the student volunteer. Although some patients apparently tried to maintain the "sick" role, this was embarrassing to others. One student also noticed a role change in patients when they were returned to the hospital attendants. This problem, elaborated in greater detail later in the chapter, was a constant source of difficulty in the program. The student also began setting goals for herself and her group.

DORIS: *I have noticed also that Martha depressed the whole group. It is as if she is showing me how sick people can be. Whenever I ask her anything, the group tenses up, hoping that she won't give their secrets away. In addition, there was a complete change in the group when the attendant came. They suddenly became expres-*

sionless robots again. It seems as if they have no pride, hopes, individuality or happiness. I wonder if seeing me doesn't depress them further. I may be able to please them for one hour on Thursday, but what about the rest of the time? If these people even wanted to get out of the hospital, who would they turn to for support?

I am looking forward to the next session with mixed feelings. I hope to get some enthusiasm out of them one of these days. Actually, if I can just make them happy with themselves, I will feel as if I have accomplished quite a bit!

The last and most lengthy excerpt from the initial reactions serves as a good summary of the feelings many students had about their first group meeting. It also provides several interesting descriptions of patients, both within the group and in the hospital at large. Finally, it sounds a note of apprehension for the task lying ahead.

DONALD: *After going through much anxiety I managed to survive to face the group tonight. I never felt any fear about what would happen, only fear about what might not. I went in armed with my bingo set which I hoped I wouldn't have to use. The moment of truth arrived and I entered the barren room with the hardest chairs I'd ever seen scattered about. I was presented with my first two patients, Jim and Larry. Larry was small and frail and was exactly as I pictured Billy Bibbit in"One Flew Over the Cuckoo's Nest" I'd almost guess that they came from the same type of background. Larry would talk about a good many things when prompted, so I took advantage of this and tried to find out a little more about the place. Jim was quite large, breathed very heavily and smoked continuously. He was the first person I'd ever seen roll a cigarette. He did this while one was still lit. He didn't say much and seemed very tired and sluggish and gave the impression of being heavily drugged. In came two more after a while, Carl and William. Carl was probably the oldest in the group and possibly the most intelligent. He seemed more aware of what was happening in the outside world than the others. Will was dressed in white and I gathered he worked in the kitchen which turned out to be correct. He seemed quite agreeable to almost everything and said he liked to sketch. Last to come was Bruce, a Negro, who also seemed to be quite heavily sedated, in addition to being rather reserved. All five would respond to anything I asked and on a couple of occasions they responded to each other. They didn't often offer anything without prompting, and they had to be addressed by name to get a response.*

I got the feeling that they had all come from similar backgrounds, namely lower class, and had received only a minimum of education. I'm sure several didn't finish high school even though we didn't discuss that at all. I would guess they weren't able to find steady jobs and couldn't find satisfaction in our society, so they dropped out.—Here they are and here they'll stay . . .

The most evident characteristic that I saw was apathy. This place seems to breed it on both sides of the fence. These men don't give a damn about anything—but why should they? After 10-15 years of this, we don't have the right to expect them to feel differently. I get the feeling that each one could have been helped more when they first came to the hospital and maybe they wouldn't be there today.

I tried to find what they like to do. Larry likes games (monopoly) and records and Westerns on television. Carl likes to read; he gets "Life." William likes to paint. Bruce couldn't get too enthusiastic over anything.

Frequently they would talk of things they used to do, but don't do any more. Jim used to work and go to occupational therapy, but no more. Carl had a job but his ward was changed and he can't work any more. They said the hospital used to use more patients to do jobs like baking bread, etc., but these have all stopped.

I wish I could think that what I'm doing will be of some help, but I can't quite conceive of it. The hospital has done such a good job of dehumanization that no one could quite overcome it. I don't necessarily say that they would improve in a different atmosphere, but I'm sure they won't in this one. I still have the fear that I won't know what to do with them week after week and that I will quickly get discouraged with the whole thing. There's no turning back, though, so I can only wait and see.

X. PATIENT GROUP MEETINGS

As patient meetings proceeded over the year, occurrences in each group were determined by many factors, some anticipated, some not. The group format, that established certain broad limits, is not necessarily a part of college-student volunteer programs. Indeed, most prior programs have been based on a one-to-one format. For this and other programs the choice between group or individual contacts is an important decision. Each has advantages and disadvantages, and depending on the particular situation, a reasoned choice must be made.

In the one-to-one arrangement, a group of students is typically introduced to a ward and the individual student is largely free to work with one or several patients of his choice. In such a situation, the student has the advantage of focusing his time and energy on a single patient. A disadvantage of the one-to-one interaction is that it does not promote patient-peer contact. Group meetings emphasizing patient interaction may thus generalize more readily to the everyday activities of the target group, particularly if ward staff is incorporated into the program. For patients who are about to be released, developing a relation with a single student—a "significant other" from the community—may be useful in combating recidivism. If the volunteer can follow the patient after his discharge, he can continue to serve as a "significant other" within the community. For chronic patients still far from being released, focusing on the group process may be more useful. Whereas we did not wish to be defeatists on the matter of patient discharge, we did want to be realists. The discharge rate for chronic patients at the Rochester State Hospital has always been very low. Moreover, since that variable was not within our control, hospital discharge policy was likely to remain the same.

In this project, the group arrangement was chosen for several reasons. The most important and practical of these was the need to limit the number of volunteers so that we could provide adequate supervision. Concern about adequate supervision cannot be passed over lightly. As more colleges and universities establish volunteer programs (frequently student initiated), and as more settings accept such programs, there is the danger that the issue of adequate supervision can be lost. While programs may legitimately range from technique-oriented behavior modification types to those that harness natural interpersonal skills, and "nonprofessionalness" of volunteers, all require continuing close contact with a "guiding force." Supervision, at the very least, provides a mechanism for communication with, and continued feedback to, volunteers, and a forum for their own role-concerns. Without this, volunteers stand to lose perspective and motivation. The problem of dropouts can reach significant proportions, and the sense of purpose and clinical responsibility for constructive patient change, can be lost in diffuse "do-gooder" notions. When volunteers perceive themselves as seen by the hospital staff and by patients as bona fide helping persons, rather than as "time-fillers," their potential for usefulness increases. This matter takes on growing importance as service programs rapidly expand. Institutions sponsoring such programs must provide on-going supervision if the programs are to succeed.

Our wish to include as large a patient sample as possible was another reason for using a group format. Moreover, we were interested, theoretically, in group processes in patient–patient and patient–student interaction. Finally, we were dealing with chronic patients who were not immediate candidates for release from the hospital and were likely to spend much time back on the wards. Lacking skills needed for small group interaction, it seemed likely that they would continue, passively, to ignore one another. Thus, with the simultaneous aims of increasing social skills in chronic hospitalized patients, extending the scope of the program, and maximizing research potential, we decided to have group meetings.

While the group format has the above-mentioned advantages, its nature is such that the student-leader is but one member of a multiperson situation. He faces not only the challenge of establishing a relationship between himself and eight patients, but also other demands intrinsic to the group format (e.g., conflict between members). Moreover, he has no choice as to the group with which he will work.

The use of small rooms off the wards necessarily limited some activities (e.g., physical ones) and predisposed toward others (e.g., table games). Again, an arbitrary choice was made, since the groups could have met on the ward. Although doing so might conceivably have promoted generalization of positive effects, it would also have created several insuperable drawbacks. Beyond the fact that the design required control patients from the same wards who continued in the normal hospital routine, there were other advantages to using off-ward meeting rooms. These rooms became "special" to many patients. Since overcrowded hospital living conditions allowed for little or no privacy, the meeting rooms were seen as a separate place, belonging to the patients, and away from hospital routine. As interpersonal cohesiveness increased, the groups often took on the quality of semiautonomous units. Many patients referred to the groups as "clubs." The meeting room served as a kind of "clubhouse."

Many group activities centered on improving the physical conditions of the meeting rooms. For example, as noted previously, one rather frail coed was seen carrying a huge rug over her shoulder. She brought the rug in to make the room feel "warmer." During group sessions, curtains were made and walls were decorated with posters, paintings, and sketches. Indeed, occasional problems developed when staff removed such items, but eventually an understanding was reached that the meeting rooms would not be disturbed. Some positive changes in patient behavior (e.g., greater outgoingness and broader perspective) were doubtless furthered by allowing them to meet in a separate off-ward place and to encounter different role-expectations from those experienced on the ward.

At the same time, the use of the off-ward meeting rooms probably limited the generalization of newly acquired skills and responses to the ward. Marked changes from within-meeting behavior to behavior outside the room were continually, and clearly, in evidence. Patients often came out of the group meetings beaming and excitedly holding some object made in the group, that now *belonged* to them. Within moments, however, the stark hospital atmosphere and the unimpressed glares of attendants transformed the initial flush of enthusiasm to the more typical dull, apathetic expressions that these patients normally presented on the ward.

One student-leader from an afternoon group, Penny, who met her patients at the ward door, commented:

> *One thing that we've all noticed is the change in the patients when they come to the meetings and when they go to the wards. June is a perfect example. I pick her up at the ward and she looks really depressed and barely says anything. She obediently stands at the elevator and follows everyone downstairs, etc. When we're in the room, she smiles and jokes and talks about her family and enjoys herself. But as soon as I say, "Well, it's time to go," she turns off and becomes the same lethargic, docile being she was before. I don't think anyone is going to see any changes in them except us . . .*
>
> *I was also teaching Mary how to knit. She did three stitches and looked up at me beaming. But she can't take the needles back to the ward because they're too sharp. Ugh!*

Another limitation of the meeting-room arrangement was that it focused away from outside activities such as trips to the community for shopping or recreational events. Although there were several rehearsal-type discussions of what patients might do "downtown" in a store, there was no opportunity to practice, *in vivo*, these independent social activities. Actually, this problem was not solely due to using off-ward meeting rooms; it also reflected a lack of administrative sanction for outside semiautonomous activities by the student–patient groups.

When groups were grudgingly allowed to go outside the building during the final third of the program, for the most part they had to remain in fenced-in portions of the grounds adjoining the buildings. A very few trips to the hospital bowling alleys permitted during the last weeks of the program, were major events for the patients and stimulated great excitement.

Within the framework of these restrictions, there was considerable variety in group activities. Student-leaders were not limited to the verbal format of traditional therapy groups. Many of the group activities developed during the program highlight the helping potential of nonprofessionals. Indeed, the wide variety of activities per se highlights the tremendous flexibility of the nonprofessional role. Some activities revealed particular skills of student leaders, such as playing a musical instrument or a knowledge of photography. Some indicated a great deal of originality. One group leader initiated role-playing techniques by having the group enact hisotrical scenes:

PAULA: *I brought a camera and we were taking pictures about great moments in history, for example, King Henry VIII giving the signal for the executioner to behead Anne Boleyn. It was cute. Catherine was the executioner, wielding a crochet hook. I said, "Catherine, why don't you be the executioner?" She made a placating face and said, "Oh, I'll do it or you'll tease me until you get your way." But you could tell that she wanted to do it.*

The patients attached great importance to food. Students learned quickly that food was a major incentive for group attendance and interaction. For females, this interest included both preparing and eating food. Most students brought some kind of food, often homemade, with them each week. Cigarettes were also found to be a meaningful commodity. Many group games used food, cigarettes, or both as prizes.

One group demonstrated free-enterprise in action by setting up a "cigarette manufacturing company." Each group member participated in rolling cigarettes. These were sold by the patients during the week and some proceeds went toward more cigarette materials, while profits were used to supply treats for the group members.

Despite variability in specific group activities, a high premium was, throughout, placed on patient interaction. Many students sought to promote spontaneous and "leaderless" group discussions. Improved patient interaction was often noted as in the following excerpt:

BILL: *It gets easier all the time for me to be just talking with them. I also care less about silences. Max has shown, for him, a remarkable upsurge in politeness, cheerfulness, and alertness towards me . . . . He greets me when he comes in and responds much more nicely when asked to join us, although he still refuses. Last time, he actually initiated a brief conversation!*

The last comment in this excerpt highlights the student-leaders' efforts to elicit responses from noncommunicative patients. Active communication in previously nonresponsive patients occurred frequently, though not always in the dramatic form of the monopoly game incident cited in Chapter 1. Such moments were exciting to the volunteers. The following excerpt both illustrates new-found patient responsiveness and reflects an attribute of many leaders—unmitigated enthusiasm:

DORIS: *Headway was made with Martha today. Yahoo!!!! She laughed with me, and I even got her to play Bingo. Will wonders never cease? The nurse said that she hasn't seen Martha make any type of attempt to associate with anyone for 20 years. This makes it all worth it!!! Will have to try some more on Tuesday!*

While specific techniques were not systematically taught to students, and the program emphasized their "natural" social reflexes, some did in fact apply behavior-control techniques, typically a derivative of behavior modification methodology. Modeling of prosocial behavior and role playing were frequent. Students were advised in discussions sessions, to be consistent, to ignore deviant behavior, and to reinforce, through attention, positive behavior. An example is noted in one student's diary:

PATRICIA: *Dick came in as usual and asked for his cigarette before he sat down to silently smoke away the hour. I wanted him to call me by name and not call me "Dick," which is his name. He calls everyone "Dick." It went like this:*

"I want you to use my name. My name is Patricia."
"Give me a couple of cigarettes."
"What's my name?"
"I don't know."
"My name is Patricia."
"Give me a couple of cigarettes, Dick."

This went on for a few minutes until he finally used my name! Later Dick asked for another cigarette. I asked him once to use my name and he did. So I gave him the cigarette. A little progress!?

Experiences such as this were fairly common. Sometimes, especially during the first few weeks, students were astonished by the bizarreness of patient behavior. In one case, a cigarette that a student offered to a patient was promptly eaten. In another, the supervisor suggested that a student bring modeling clay to his group. The student sheepishly explained that this had already been tried, but rather than using the clay for modeling, the patient ate it! For the most part, however, students met patients with the expectation that they would behave in a "normal" manner. More often than not, the patient's behavior, at least during the group meetings, changed to meet such expectations.

"Breakthroughs" frequently occurred when the patient was put into a position of responsibility. However minor this responsibility may have seemed to the casual observer, it was often far more than had previously been given by hospital staff. The following example illustrates the point:

PENNY: *We . . . put popcorn up to pop. Eve kept getting up and going over to look and see if it was popping. I said, "Eve's going to be our official popcorn popper watcher." Then shock of shocks, she said something completely intelligible. I felt terrible because I didn't know what to say to her . . . but I was really pleased that she had finally spoken spontaneously. The other patients looked more surprised than I because they had kept telling me that she never talks.*

Many activities were specifically related to the sex of the leader and group members. Groups with male patients and male students were more interested in physical activities. Female patients with female students spent a lot of time on grooming activities, such as polishing nails and setting each other's hair. Many female patients wore new hairstyles; some combed their hair for the first time in years. Indeed, a number were upset when male student leaders did not notice these changes.

The particular effectiveness of the female student–male patient groups, noted in our research data, was also apparent observationally. Interactions in these groups most closely resembled what might be considered "dating" behavior. Changes in male patients exemplifying this behavior reflected the "awakening process" described in Chapter 5. There was a notable increase in concern about personal cleanliness and dress. During the first weeks of the program, when the authors themselves brought the patients to the meetings, incontinent males were not infrequently found lying on the floor in urine stenched clothes. Seeing these same patients three months later, dressed and shaved for a meeting, was truly a dramatic experience. The sight of one male patient wearing a wide flowered tie and checked flannel shirt, with his hair slicked back and a broad smile revealing a missing front tooth, was among the handsomest pictures we saw during the program.

Two excerpts from the diaries of female students who worked with male patients describe their experience from this perspective:

KATY: *Bowling—on the walk over, Dave said, "It's nice to be free again, at least a little." Claude and Jim were dressed in jackets and ties and looked really good. What was most fantastic was Jake. He hadn't done anything all year, and he bowled today and got the best score of anyone. Dan started out really happy, but when he couldn't bowl well, he began getting angry and upset and lapsed into his mumbling about how bad sex is, etc. John gave me a compact that he had found somewhere. Jim was really friendlier than usual and seemed to enjoy bowling very much. He said it was much better than the games we usually play—he did fantastically well considering he never bowled before. They also liked the soda I brought, so I'll have to do that again, too. We stayed for an extra half hour so we could play two games. Everyone improved and everyone seemed to enjoy it. A definite must again if possible.*

A second student underscores the "dating" reaction:

BEATRICE: Personal appearance must be commented on. Mel asked about my rings and everyone examined them. He also asked if I had gotten a haircut, which made me realize I had my hair "up" for the first time since I had been coming. This seemed to start Harry thinking, because he kept eyeing me with a pleased look on his face. When I teasingly asked what he was looking at, he said "I'm just admiring your good looks." I said I was flattered, etc., and he went on to talk about my eyelashes. I said kiddingly that if he kept this up I'd be sure to put him down at the other end of the table and he equally good-humoredly assured me that he "wasn't trying to get fresh." He has lately begun to talk about girlfriends he used to have, and tonight he mentioned a wife.

In several groups, patients treated the students in a maternal or a paternal fashion. In others, patients treated the students as peers. Many groups reflected the beneficial effects of closeness in role-status between the student nonprofessional and patient. The building of strong trusting relationships between students and patients is one such example. The development of trust was a reciprocal process. Students were genuinely happy when the patients cared about them, as for example, when patients asked if they would return next week. Patients seemed equally gratified and, for many, such concern was unique, not having been felt, or at least observably so, for many years previously. The building of trust was quite exemplified in sharing personal experiences. Most often students initiated this process, thus, serving as a model for self-disclosure:

BILL: After revealing personal information—about the death of a close relative . . . we talked about this a little more, and they were very understanding and sympathetic. I doubted for a minute whether I should bring the subject up, but decided to be frank with them as I always have been. They responded quite appropriately I thought, and perhaps it was good for them to have a chance to feel sorry for someone else and not themselves.

Sometimes it was the patient who initiated the disclosure process:

TED: Barry revealed a little about his past drinking habits—noting how bad they were. I was rather impressed that he spoke so freely of his past—it was the first time he had ever done so. For this reason, I, too, revealed a little about my personal life; I mentioned my father's untimely death and its effects upon the family.

Perceived closeness in the social status hierarchy and the flexibility of the nonprofessional facilitated identification between patient and student. Occasionally such closeness was uncomfortable for the latter:

PENNY: *While we were cleaning up, Mary came over to me and said, "I wish I were more like you." I said, "Why, wouldn't you rather be yourself? You're pretty, etc." She said, "No, I'd rather be like you." I tried to convince her that it was better to be oneself and I touched her face, gently, to show that I understood. She flinched. This whole episode really made me feel helpless. She came in with a desperate pleading in her voice and I could tell her nothing to ease it. I sympathized and offered suggestions, but it all seemed so futile.*

This incident, and others like it, also reflect an awareness of some of the hopelessness of the patients' situation. Some students were genuinely depressed when they became aware of this. One student, for example, noted:

DON: *One night Sam began to shake and kept demanding to go back to the ward, saying he thought he was going to faint. I went downstairs for the attendant, who sneered when I told him. After a long wait he came up and as he took Sam into the ward I heard:*

Sam: "I ain't feeling so good."
Attendant: "Aw, you ain't been good for years."

It's like banging your head against a wall. I've had this nausea about the hospital an awful lot lately. I never used to, but just now, coupled with complete discouragement, it's started up. These people are rotting.

Another student reported:

PENNY: *As I was walking into the building, a group of men gathered by the windows called out. The sight of them locked up as in a cage, trying to attract attention, really depressed me. Quite often I try to view my men in terms of our group meetings, as isolated from the rest of their depressing existence. The men at the window make their helplessness more real to me.*

These instances quite naturally served to temper students' expectations about their own effectiveness. They also increased their indignation toward the hospital. As noted in the attitude-change data reported in Chapter 6, students came, as a result of their program participation, to view the hospital less favorably. The same experiences did not, however, lead to rejection of patients. On the contrary, they fostered even greater acceptance of them, and of the belief that patient problems did not simply reflect a "disease" but rather were an inevitable product of their social situation:

TED: *Barry wasn't there again. He's barricaded himself in the seclusion room; he refused to eat or drink and refused medication as well. They had to give him shots. He didn't want to see his parents and struck them when he did. I asked whether or not I could see him. The attendant said, "No visitors!" It's really pretty depressing especially since Barry is about the best patient I have. The attendant said maybe he would be back next week—maybe not though, too. I almost can't picture him being violent and uncooperative as they say he is now. He's always seemed so normal, so much like a regular good guy. How can he react as he is? It seems nearly impossible to me!*

It's funny. This whole episode with Barry has made me realize that these patients are very much human beings. Yet the life—or shall I say the existence—they lead is a very sad state of affairs. What do they live for? Have they what may be properly called a "life?" It seems more of a prison term with no hope of reprieve. No wonder they all seem apathetic to everything. I would too if I existed in a building without even being allowed to go outside and walk around by myself. Privacy? Individuality? These words swim around in my mind—what do they mean to the patients?

A description of the patients and of group meetings should not overlook the fact that there were also moments of light-heartedness and humor. Indeed, frequently it was only the good sense of humor of the students that allowed them to continue in the program. (The same might also be said of the authors.)

The following excerpt recounts one of the humorous situations:

PENNY: *Then I mentioned LSD and tried to explain what it was. I told them a story about a boy at Columbia who thought he saw a beautiful lake and jumped, but he was actually jumping 10 floors down onto the pavement. Millie said, "Did he die?" I said, "Yes." She said, "Then how did they know what he saw?" A pretty quick response, which I had trouble talking my way out of.*

A second excerpt is a tongue-in-cheek prescription for dealing with a patient who constantly spoke of religious fantasies:

BILL: *You see, the formula goes like this. If you start any type of discussion with Frank, on any subject, it takes about three minutes before he manipulates it into a matter of religion. Therefore, if you switch to a new subject about every 2½ minutes, you can avoid this. If you wait 3 to 3½ minutes, you will find that Frank becomes engrossed in his end of the discussion and he will not stop talking about it, even if you've moved on to something else.*

About midway through the program, it was clear that in order for the students to continue to bring food, cigarettes and various supplies to the hospital, as they had done to that point, some financial support was necessary. The project, although it involved over 320 patients, 32 volunteers, eight to ten graduate students and three or four undergraduate assistants, was operating on a precarious total budget of less than $5000. Under those circumstances it was impossible to find money for food or supplies, so that the students were spending an average of $1 to $2 each, per week, for such things. When it became obvious that many students could no longer afford the financial strain, the authors appealed to a university service fraternity and were given $600 for supplies.

As the program moved into high gear, a variety of affects and changes could be identified in the student leaders: depression, anger, pleasure, and some satisfaction; a growing respect for the patients, and an increasing sophistication and wordliness about the hospital maze. Few students were apathetic about any aspect of the experience. On the contrary, the project was highly meaningful to all. Of the 32 original volunteers, only two were so uncomfortable with the situation that they asked to drop out. These students, one male and one female, both terminated after the first several meetings. Each felt that he could not comfortably work with his patient group. The other 30 students maintained generally appropriate levels of anxiety, and demonstrated a high degree of clinical responsibility. Even when they were personally very busy, or having a difficult time in school, they maintained patient responsibility. As one student put it:

MARY: *It's funny. I was fully expecting a lousy session. The past week has been hell for me. Finals always make me realize how little oriented to academia I am, and my schedule has the appearance of a devil's plot. Sleep seemed to have disappeared from life. So I brought coffee (forgetting milk, which amused but didn't daunt my people) and borrowed Dick's popcorn popper. I told them how it was, and a conversation was started about school.*

We started a ping-pong tournament and Mr. Baker, Mr. Ford, and Mr. Stone won their matches. I'll have to bring in a map of the wins next Wednesday.

Mr. Baker in particular talked about the hospital a lot—he was on a closed ward for 20 years where they had to scrub floors to earn a bag of tobacco to roll a few cigarettes per day. Food was awful. He escaped (left) twice and the police caught him. He must have been in the hospital for about 30 or more years. He and Eddie see the changes in the hospital, better food, more leniency.

Someone, an old man who was in at least 30 years, died Sunday.

Fred mentioned that in spring he may go to the V.A. hospital. It was like discussing any move, damn it, because he seems so normal and pleasant.

What was so great about the session was that they showed initiative. Not in actually doing something so much as in acting as though I were not there to organize and entertain, I was just visiting.

Mr. Jones asked if I ever became tired because of my coming to be with them. That seemed so nice of him, to think that I was inconvenienced. He also mentioned suddenly beginning to scream at our last session, and he got all excited suddenly. I didn't pursue it because I knew he could bring it up again.

For the first time I didn't feel obligated to be an activities counselor. I was there as a person, as me.

The University of Rochester has not been immune to the feelings of unrest so widely encountered today among college students. Cries for "relevance" on campus echo as loudly there as they do in most other institutions of higher learning. The wish to make academic life more directly relevant to the "real world" is not uncommon among Rochester's undergraduates. During the project year, there were a number of antiwar demonstrations on campus. About two-thirds of the way through the program, in protest against an on-campus recruiter from a chemical company making weapons materials used in Viet Nam, there was a general strike at the University. Almost all of our student-leaders participated in this strike. To our surprise and satisfaction, however, they all continued to attend patient and supervisory meetings. Many voiced the opinion that, "This is different; this is the kind of relevance we are asking for!" In some ways, this incident was more meaningful to us as an index of the "significance" of the program to student leaders than were many of the formal research findings.

XI. THE "SPECIAL" GROUP

At this point, we should consider the unique contribution of one student, Bill, in Psychology 278. When Bill responded initially to the announcement of the proposed practicum, questions arose about how he might be used. He is blind. After our screening interview with him, however, we decided that he was qualified, both educationally and personally, to participate. An issue that came up in our preliminary discussion was whether he should have direct responsibility for profoundly ill, chronic, hospitalized patients. We considered placing him in the elementary school project, but his preference was for the hospital program. We discussed the matter openly with him, and were persuaded that Bill was indeed capable of handling the considerable demands of the hospital situation. We were not incorrect.

For research purposes, it was not possible to include him in the main study. We decided instead to use him in the acute treatment unit, where he was put in charge of a "special" group of hospitalized adolescents. The group included youngsters who refused to talk to their physician, and others who were suicidal, withdrawn, hostile, or angry. According to reports, both from patients and from the ward psychiatrist, Bill was "a phenomenal success." Some staff members who did not know him inquired about the "new psychologist." Adolescents who had been transferred to other wards asked to continue attending Bill's group sessions. Bill himself stayed in Rochester during his Christmas vacation in order to continue patient contacts.

Although Bill's strikingly positive impact was, in good measure, due to his high-level interpersonal skills, he also engendered the feeling in adolescent patients that their problems were minimal compared to his. At the same time, Bill was able to "model" efficient coping behavior. Bill went on to enroll in a Ph.D. clinical psychology program at a major university. Below are transcribed some of his observations, kept on a tape-recorded diary:

> *I wish I had a tape recorder tonight. People were talking about their experiences and responding to each other. This session was the most worthwhile one so far. The patients were all extremely open and I really felt that I helped them. I felt that I pointed many things out to them and that they accepted some of the things that I said. Probably what makes these sessions so worthwhile is that people have the opportunity to talk about things that are bothering them. The patients claim that they talk about things here that they don't even tell the psychiatrist. There must be a lot of trust within the group, and with me. The greatest feeling on my part is that I*

am contributing something. I feel I am more aware of what the patients need and also what they might want to give to me . . . .

Well, it's all over and I still have mixed emotions about it. I really wonder how much they benefited by coming there twice a week. There's no doubt in my mind that a lot of these patients did improve, but who knows what the cause is? Probably the biggest thing in their favor was time. But to say the least, I feel that this course was one of the most valuable courses that I have taken at this university and all that I can say as far as the 15 or 20 patients that I did see is maybe I did help one of them in some way.

XII. TERMINATION

Termination was discussed extensively both in the student–supervisor and patient groups. The reactions of students and patients were like those of persons being separated from good friends. For some patients, termination of the program marked the end of the first friendship they had experienced in many years and many were upset about that. Some instances of reawakening of discarded serious symptoms were reported, but these were exceptions rather than the rule. The single most common patient concern was the hope that the program might continue when the students returned in the fall.

The students felt they had worked hard over the course of 5½ months and many were looking foward to graduating. Although they were concerned and sad about "their" patients, they were generally realistic about termination. Most realized that despite their efforts, many patients would remain in the hospital; they had come to accept this. They were reconciled to the fact that, for a brief while, they had offered some patients an oasislike change from their usual flat hospital life and had shared a portion of their own lives with them. Where patients had relearned social skills that could enrich even their ward life, that was an important accomplishment. Many students continued to visit patients after the program ended and some were still corresponding with them two years later. Typical termination reactions from student diaries are presented below:

JOHN: *The meeting was particularly ordinary but I was conscious of time almost exactly like I was at the first few meetings. I found myself looking for changes in the people and they were there in subtle ways—considering others in the distribution of food, saying thank you and things like that. John also seemed more open in his conversation. To an outside observer the changes might go unnoticed but being involved as I was the little changes were important. We all shook hands at the end but I think only John was aware that the groups were over.*

Another student wrote:

MARY: *I'm really dreading the end. Even though I haven't always wanted to come or done my best, I have learned a lot about the hospital and my patients. I wish there were some way to expose everyone to the hospital so the stereotypes would disappear. My dream is a grade school program continued through high school orienting all students, especially non-college bound to community service . . .*

A bird flew in our room—what a funny thing to happen on our last day. Everyone wants to know if the program will go next year.

It's a different kind of committment, this program. No one pushes really, just 8 patients who look forward to your coming. A much "realer" thing than academia.

The attendant told me something of Mr. Smith's life. He used to work for the Post Office. That's frightening— my father does and he is like Mr. Smith sometimes. Anyway, he had a wife and kids. They told him his wife had a new baby—and he hasn't been at home in longer than that—and the attendant said he didn't even seem to care.

I'll miss them—just as people I met and became involved with—some I liked and its all very sad.

The final excerpt cited below makes general observations on society, and points up the most disappointing aspect of the program:

SUSAN: *I am starting to feel bad now that it's over. Not that I feel that I've done so much for them—but they all have such unique personalities that they've all made a definite impression. I also feel pretty badly about not having done more. Not so much as far as activities, I just would've liked to make things a little more hopeful for them. But I'm still able to walk out of there in a week and they have to stay there and vegetate. Marge's written me a few poems in the interim. Really interesting although not good aesthetically. All of them repeatedly tell me to find the answer. She's much more of a mystery than the others—even knowing her history wouldn't help too much I think. The one who bothers me most is Joan . . . she's really a great person and I know somehow she'll never get out of there for one reason or another. She really doesn't belong there, When I first met her she was just apathetic, but who wouldn't be after a few years in that place. Alice is really a sad case—she won't even try to help herself—but why go on—it's really pathetic and one person is pretty much inadequate. The one conclusion I have reached is that our society is basically primitive or spartanic in its approach to "different" people. Shutting abnormal human beings out of the world doesn't solve anything; but why go on?*

It was difficult, but not impossible, for student leaders to accept the fact that some patients would remain in the hospital. Most also believed the groups had been valuable to patients. What was hardest to accept, however, was the realization that many patients who had made so much progress during the year would have to remain in the hospital simply because they had no other place to go. These "marginal" individuals could have functioned outside hospital walls if the social system could have provided them a place in the world. In this matter, authors and students agreed. "In-community" settings, such as Fairweather's (1969) self-sustaining half-way house for patients, hold special promise for future programming. The possibility of combining in-hospital use of nonprofessionals to enable patients to "get ready" and community programs, also using nonprofessionals as "significant others" merits careful exploration and testing.

XIII. FAREWELL

On the Saturday following the last group meeting, a large outdoor picnic was held for all patients and student leaders who had participated in the program. The purposes of the picnic were twofold: to soften the blow of termination and to be a small reward for the heroic effort of students and staff who had contributed so much to the program.

The picnic was a tremendous success! Through donations of a university service fraternity and local merchants, there was more than enough food and treats for all 250 people who attended. Despite the festive atmosphere, however, it was a day for farewells and there were tears shed by both students and patients. Perhaps the most difficult moment for the authors occurred at the end of the picnic when the patients were once again lined up by the attendants to return to their wards. For an instant, we wondered if the program had ever really taken place.

On the day of the final supervisory meeting after the program ended—a meeting billed in highly intellectual terms as a summary and "stock-taking" meeting—the student leaders surprised the authors with a party. The party ended up in an off-campus tavern. Everyone drank a lot of beer, shared a lot of feelings, and expressed emotional relief. It is difficult, in retrospect, to pull together the full impact of a year of working so closely with undergraduates directly engaging a major problem of contemporary society. Nevertheless, the positive feeling and mutual regard expressed at that party left the authors with a considerably improved personal understanding of what meaningful undergraduate education can be.

XIV. STUDENT AND HOSPITAL REACTIONS TO OUTCOME

A formal account of program effectiveness, evaluated in terms of performance and behavior change both in groups and on the ward, has already been given. The softer aspects of the project and of patient change have been considered in the immediately preceding sections. In the section to follow, overall student and institutional reactions are reviewed.

The students were asked on the GAF to note changes in patient groups over the course of the program and to cite the reasons, if known, for such improvement. To summarize, and to illustrate some perceived patient advances, comments have been extracted from these periodic evaluations, and representative examples are presented as follows:

We are much more of a group now.

Conversation comes easier; the patients are more active and enthusiastic.

They are talking more to each other and are more at ease.

I don't have to keep them busy, there is more unity.

They are more willing to put themselves out for others.

They give me more feedback.

They trust me more.

While students and staff agreed that individual patients had benefitted from the program, an important latent goal was to model a project which, if workable, could help to move hospital administration a significant step forward on the dimension going from custodial care to active treatment. Although the program, during much of its existence, was largely peripheral to the hospital's basic functions, signs developed during its course that the dragon was at least on its feet if not yet moving. Slowly the staff came to see the program as a bit less of a nuisance and, indeed, as something of moderate interest. We noted before in illustrating this change that several groups were permitted to go outside the hospital grounds during the late phases of the program. Permission to use hospital bowling alleys was also granted. These were small but important steps.

In addition, the occupational therapy department contributed some supplies to the program. Coffee began to be supplied by the kitchen staff, and cookies for the group meetings were baked by female patients on intensive-care units. Supplies were made available by the hospital for the final picnic. In some small measure, the hospital had come to be more concerned about the well being and enjoyment of chronic patients heretofore largely ignored.

Increasingly, members of the professional staff began to ask about the program, i.e., to inquire periodically of its progress. At the end, the authors were invited to talk to the entire hospital staff about the program and its effects. Of major importance, in that it represented a first step of the dragon under its own power, was the request that the program be continued in the future, perhaps the first active step in chronic patient care taken by the hospital in many years. The college student program is, at the time of this writing, an ongoing one at the Rochester State Hospital.

XV. FOLLOW-UP INTERVIEW WITH STUDENTS

In order to obtain a better idea of how the student volunteer experience was seen in perspective about 6 months after the program ended, four student leaders were invited to discuss their impressions and reactions. These four students, two males and two females, had been juniors during the program period and were still on campus. They were selected largely because of that fact and because it was possible to bring them together as a group at a time that was free for the interviewer. There is no reason to assume that they represented anything but a random cross-section of the junior student leaders from the preceding year. The group interview, which lasted about 30 minutes, was tape recorded and is reproduced below:

INT.: *Let me start off with several general questions: "Just how do you view your experience in the undergraduate practicum last year? What do you see as its purpose and its objectives, and the ways in which it did and did not work out?"*

JOHN: *The obvious attraction for me was that it would be an opportunity for some practical experience—something I needed. This has been the only experience I've really had through 3½ years, in which I was given an opportunity to have some actual contact with people.*

SUSAN: *I agree. That's what I thought was most interesting. And I think that's what* **most** *people who took the course liked about it. It* *gave us the chance to get out into the field, and to apply, in our own ways, the things we'd been learning for three years.*

HANK: *I don't think it was mere experience. It was exposure to what was* real. *I don't think I had a chance to apply too much of any kind of psych knowledge I had. I think it was based on our relations with people and gave me a little exposure to different types of people. I really don't think there was direct application from things I learned in a textbook.*

POLLY: *I found that the most worthwhile part of this experience was exposing us to the whole field of prevention which, personally, I hadn't been aware of. I didn't know such things were going on in community groups and residential schools and it opened my eyes to new fields that I might be interested to work in. I found, working in the hospital, that I was relating to people. It was the experience I got in seeing those people that I've used since—knowing what they're like. I didn't use very much of what I'd learned in courses. Maybe it means that what you learn in psych courses really doesn't apply.*

INT.: *Well, we didn't rehearse that question and I suppose it could have been answered in either of two ways: from* your *point of view or from the patient's standpoint. Maybe we can also approach it now with that second question in mind. What do you see as the purposes of the program, centering on the patients?*

HANK: *At times I wasn't* sure *if it meant a lot to the patients, but the very fact that they kept coming back,—whether they said they enjoyed it or that it was worth anything to them—that gave at least some indication that it was worth it.*

SUSAN: *Since most of the patients we were working with were on chronic wards, many of their interactions were with other maladjusted people. The program gave them a chance to communicate with someone from the outside who could bring in new points of view—give them a little better life.*

JOHN: *I think that the experience we had emphasized the sorry state of mental health approaches and the need to do something about it* right now. *It was frustrating and aggravating at times, too. You could only go there a couple of times a week and then you're not really near it again until the next week. Yet, for these people it's a break in their day-in, day-out experience. I think it's unrealistic to expect* dramatic *improvement in a patient who has to put up with an institution of that kind—a total institution.*

POLLY: *You wonder what happens after we're gone. Five or six months of working with them, once, twice a week and then you tell them—you prepare them for a month about your leaving and then you're gone. And, I don't know of many people who have gone back and visited, no matter how much we said we might do it. I wrote during the summer but that was the summer and now you're back in class.*

INT.: *O.K.! Let's come back to things a little more concretely now. It might be helpful if each of you, in turn, would take a couple, three minutes, to describe the interaction that you and your group had, so as to give us a notion of exactly what you went through. What was the experience like and what actually happened?*

POLLY: *Well, as a group, having 6–8 men each week—I felt a real need for the men to project some masculine activity. I didn't want to sit with them and make Christmas cards, or do feminine-type things, so I tried to stress things like bowling, which worked out well, and card-playing and talking about cars. If we could get them to play ping-pong because there was a ping-pong outfit, we played that, or went bowling. All this was difficult for me. I couldn't think of enough things to do. As far as my interaction with them, I think except for three men in the group, it stayed pretty much the same and one got worse. I mean there was less and less communication with him as time went on. With about three of them, we communicated better, and I'm sorry that the experience didn't continue. But that's my fault. I didn't have time.*

HANK: *I think, as a male with female patients, this was good for them. Apparently in the hospital setting they don't have too much exposure to males in the ordinary communication sense. And I think this was very good. Mainly, I did a lot of arts and crafts things—nothing too exciting. Most of the patients in my group didn't want to do anything of a physical nature like bowling. I tried to establish multiple activities rather than one. In some cases, I let them really do what they wanted, and if they didn't have any preference, then I sort of dragged them into a general activity which I'd set up. I thought that as the term progressed, my relations with them got better—not to the point I had origi-*

nally hoped, but at least to where they were much more friendlv and, at times more open about their experiences before being hospitalized and in the hospital.

JOHN: *I tried to stay away from the arts and crafts type approach. We had a project where patients manufactured and sold cigarettes, so we did rely on some manual activity. But, I tried to stay away from arts and crafts in hopes that we would get verbalizing more quickly. This obviously caused some rather awkward moments, at times, when there was little inspiration on my part and the patients were oversedated or something. After a while, the patients expressed some real dissatisfaction with their hospital situation. That was a real step in the right direction. From being passive recipients doing just about nothing, they became people who did express some discontent. They showed signs that they really weren't happy with the way things were and they could talk it out and personalize it. And I think that, hopefully, served some purpose.*

SUSAN: *I had a group of women who didn't want to do physical or athletic things. They wanted mainly to do arts and crafts, and I used a lot of music. We had a guitar player come in once, and my mother came in once. We had a beauty parlor session. They liked that, doing each other's hair and we made jewelry. Another project they decided on was to do something for children. One of the women said she'd worked at a residential treatment center for kids. I don't know whether she did or not. So, we made stuffed animals and I took them to a settlement house. Then the women at the settlement house wrote back and thanked the group and I took pictures of the kids and their animals and showed them to the group. This gave the patients a feeling that they were doing something for someone else, which appealed to them. When I first started out, we mainly talked, but they were really quiet to begin with. But, after about ten minutes, they opened up and they did start to talk. I felt, through the year, that I was getting to know them better. Then we got to a point where they were talking and although I felt I did know them to some extent, I didn't know what I could* do *for them. I felt inept to really help them in any way except besides just be a friend. So I was a friend. What was I doing? I was seeing them twice a week and then they went back on the ward. One of my patients was very ill. I don't think she changed much during the year. Another one was very happy with the system. She talked about the dances she went to. She liked it there; she was very well satisfied. Two of the others weren't satisfied, but they kind of went along with the system. They were doing well and they would probably be leaving fairly soon. Then I had one patient who wasn't really satisfied at all. She was really upset. She didn't have many people who visited her. I had a really good relationship with her I thought. She talked and she told me a lot about her problems. I think this was the person who bothered me the most, because when I left, I felt like she had made an investment in coming to the groups, and now I was just leaving her. You know, we'd had a relationship with her I thought. She talked and she told me a lot about her problems.*

INT.: *Let me tack on a couple of other subquestions. Do any of you recall your own* initial *reaction to the group and how this changed over time?*

SUSAN: *I was very enthusiastic to begin with.*

HANK: *I was very nervous to begin with—very worried about what I could do with these people and, if I could think of enough things to do. Would I run out of ideas? That fear gradually decreased because, as the year went on, the patients brought in suggestions and I kept thinking of new things. But my initial reaction was one of a little nervousness.*

POLLY: *When I'm nervous I talk a lot and I can remember bringing up things from anywhere I could think of, just to talk. Of course they all sat there, made absolutely no movement, and just sort of rocked in their chairs. I had the experience of one guy who was using his hand as an ashtray to the point of putting his cigarettes out in his hand. I just watched this. One person who stayed in the back of the room and painted stuff, was very young and consistently swearing and getting a little cross. I wouldn't have minded if I'd known him but, I didn't know why he was doing it. He never came back either.*

JOHN: *I don't know if most of us knew what to expect. I went in with some really unrealistic goals in mind. So, I set myself up for a rather dramatic disappointment in the beginning. Perhaps this was visible to the patients but after I got a little better picture of exactly what was practical and realistic and of ways in which things could be done—that was an important adjustment for me to make.*

INT.: *Let me throw you another quickie. Do you have any feelings about how the patients perceived you initially and how the perceptions may have changed over time?*

JOHN: *I got the idea that while they were outwardly appreciative, they were also a little bit dubious about what our role was, at first.*

HANK: *I think they were a little cautious in the beginning, too. I think that was overcome very soon, when you let them know that you were only a student. I think once they really realized this they opened up a lot quicker.*

SUSAN: *At first they thought we might be associated with the staff and then as we talked more about our life as a student, they became more interested in outside things and not just in our personal activities. They were always interested in what I was going to be doing, what I did on the weekends and, then I would ask them what they'd done.*

HANK: *Once in a while though, I got reactions, even later in the year, that referred to me as this "doctor" or "professional helper." Once in a while someone would call me doctor, and someone would say "He's not a doctor, he's a student." They'd have to remind each other.*

POLLY: *Some of the students said their patients called them teacher and referred to them as "my teacher." A more interesting thing was that somebody said, "Oh, you've got us because you're taking a course and you're studying us."*

JOHN: *I found that suspicion too. I think that was best alleviated as quickly as possible. While we* were *in there in part for a course and to gain interest and experience about them that wasn't the major purpose. So that perception would be the wrong understanding.*

SUSAN *I think one of the worst things we did was the tape recording. My patients changed after that. They weren't as open with me at all, after I cut the tape.*

INT.: *Tell us a little more about what you think happened!*

SUSAN: *I think they put me back in the role of someone who was watching them, because of the tape.*

INT.: *You mean part of the establishment.*

SUSAN: *Right, right. I was seen as a professional assistant rather than just a person who was interested in them.*

HANK: *I don't think that happened with me because I'd brought in a tape recorder once before. I made it part of the activity. We talked and played games with the tape recorder. We made up stories, and it was part of just another activity.*

INT.: *As a final question or area of discussion, in a very general way, do you have impressions about the program, pro or con, pitfalls or virtues, that might be useful for people about to start on this sort of experience?*

JOHN: *I guess to reiterate what I said before, maybe it would be good if they could take a quick tour through the hospital before starting with their group.*

INT.: *You're suggesting that it would be good to become familiar with the premises and to absorb some of the shock of first exposure to the hospital?*

JOHN: *Yeh, I think anything that will make your expectations a little more realistic is good. It's kind of a let-down to walk in to a dungeon-like atmosphere, and then see your ladies or your men herded down in a group on a big elevator. Even just the smell of the place needs getting used to. Walking in and handling a group are stimuli you're just not used to ordinarily. It's especially rough when you believe that something can be done, in an immediate sense. I was really kind of put down when I got there, when I saw the physical setup and the patients, and the way they were treated.*

POLLY: *I think I agree. But I'm wondering just how much effect that would have on people if they're really interested. If you're really interested and you went beforehand, how much effect would that have on your decision to go into the course? You can't really tell until you start working with your patients.*

HANK: *On a practical level, maybe it's a little efficient once you finally get into it. You know exactly, or at least you have a better idea of, what you're getting into.*

POLLY: *Or even see the room you'll be working in, so you'll know if you have a record player, if it's available.*

HANK: *Well, didn't we do that?*

POLLY: *Not the rooms we'd actually use.*

HANK: *Didn't we have a tour of the hospital, like a week before we started?*

POLLY: *But you didn't know where you'd be meeting patients personally. You just sort of oriented yourself, generally.*

SUSAN: *I think you should have two or three activities planned, too, the first time for you might feel more comfortable. And bring a snack—they like to eat!*

INT.: *Did all of you find that?*

SUSAN: *They all like to eat.*

HANK: *I think it would be good to possibly go up on the wards beforehand and meet the attendants also. Just to have a general background of what patients are talking about. If they do talk about their situation on the ward, you'll know which ward they're on, where it is, who the attendant is because a number of times they talked about their attendants and I hadn't the faintest idea who they were.*

INT.: *In almost all of the groups I sat in on last year, some students were fighting the question of how to engage these people, how to get them to interact. Was that part of your experience? And if so, did you find things that were useful to you in helping you to establish contact—meaningful contact with the patient?*

POLLY: *I think if you have a really quiet group, you might try a game activity, a table game like bingo, once—just to kind of get rapport and to learn the physical surroundings. Then try to do something to get them to interact. Just ask them questions.*

JOHN: *I think they're more comfortable when they know one another. I think that's a big help.*

SUSAN: *When I started out, I asked them about the hospital. I said I knew nothing about it and I was really interested. Like what did they have for breakfast? Did they like the food? What activities did they have? And just got their different opinions, individually–not necessarily things they're going to talk back and forth on. I think you'll find first they won't talk much at all, then they'll talk to you, and then eventually, towards the end, they start interacting. But, it takes a long time. They don't know each other either. They're all strangers. They're not from the same wards.*

JOHN: *I think we've already said you can always talk about yourself too. I think they're interested. You know, there's always something you can say about yourself.*

POLLY: *And you have to remember all through this that normal social processes take these patients ten times as long as it takes people or students who are used to that sort of thing. Maybe it would take you an hour. But it takes them a long time to learn how to trust.*

HANK: *I think you should also be aware of the ones who are a little more quiet. I found out that ones who are fairly active in the beginning are relatively happy. Compared to the others, they're always doing things, and when they didn't want to do things they could talk. But there were two or three in my group who hardly said anything and even when I asked questions, it was "I don't care" or "yes" or "no"–but nothing more. And, one should make an effort to involve these people in activities even more than the others, because the others can sort of help themselves. And, often I found that these people who don't talk as much, who don't have preferences, will participate anyway and will enjoy it. But* they *don't think so, at the beginning. And, I think an effort should be made to draw these people in.*

SUSAN: *I think the best way to engage this type person properly is to ask an objective type question. Not something that's a value judgment on their part. Simple questions were the best, like: "Would you help me with the coffee?" or "What's your favorite cookie?"–questions like that. Just to get them talking in the beginning.*

HANK: *Too often I got "I don't care" as an answer which is very hard to deal with. The "I don't care" answer leaves you where you started. You have to make some kind of decision for them. More often than not, I think you should say, "Yes, do this!" or "Help me!" rather than to say, "Well, o.k!"*

JOHN: *I think that's well put because it's a lot easier to ignore these people than it is to keep at them. And there is a tendency for some patients to go along with the people who are more out-spoken or who want to take a bigger part in the session. I think it's like Hank said, it takes a real effort to keep more or less withdrawn patients going and to help them feel they're part of the group.*

HANK: *Parallel to this, I think it should be mentioned that when people talk, it's often those who have talked all along. And a great pitfall,*

I found, is that when I talked to the members as a whole, I got answers back from just a few and the rest were passive observers. And if one isn't aware of this right from the beginning, it's very easy to think the whole group is doing something.

INT.: *Well, apropos of anything we've discussed up to this point or anything else you can think about it, if there's something you'd like to add to the record, we'd be delighted to hear from you.*

SUSAN: *I think it's probably the best experience I've had in college so far, and I really got to know myself last year.*

HANK: *I think something more can be done, although I don't have any specific recommendations. I felt that it was worthwhile, but I think, somehow in the back of my mind, there could be something even better. But, I can't put my finger on it.*

JOHN: *I think if there are some better things, one of them is sustaining the interest in the experience. We just didn't have that opportunity because of the end of the semester. Whether we would have taken advantage of it or not I don't know. But, I think there should be some outlet for continuing the program. I think it's something a larger part of the community could take part in—not just college students. There may be other untapped resources to sustain programs of this type which might be worthwhile investigating.*

INT.: *Well, I thank you all very much.*

The preceding transcript involves only a small fraction of the student leaders and their retrospective views of the program. At the same time its content, along several dimensions, reflects prevailing sentiments of many students in the program. There is no feeling of wholesale cure of patients. Rather, the program seems to have helped some patients, in modest ways, to find a little more meaningfulness in life and to establish closer contacts with the outside. The difficulties experienced by leaders in establishing meaningful contact with patients and the resourcefulness of their attempts to do so, are also apparent. One can clearly see their sense of concern about the unfortunate living conditions of the state hospital, and the adverse effects of these conditions on people exposed to them. The worth of the experience to the student leaders is frequently emphasized, although it is not always justified in terms of positive patient change. Finally, there is continued concern about the future human condition of the patients and students' feeling of regret, if not guilt, that patient contact necessarily terminated with the semester's end.

In several respects, this follow-up interview with students points up an easily overlooked byproduct of utilizing mental health volunteers. Although only indirectly a function of patient and student change, such programming, independent of its actual effectiveness, involves the local community in its own mental health services. From a public health view this is good public education. First-hand acquisition of experience and a realistic perspective on mental health and illness, the nature of large state mental hospitals, and associated educational and personal growth for participants, have considerable potential value for society. Participants are doubtless far better able, as a consequence, to act as sympathetic relatives and as informed citizens. Some leaders have gone on directly to mental health careers, others have done so less directly, but even those who did not are more competent in their understanding of mental health issues as they relate to their own families and to the public at large. This type of experience is potentially open to hundreds of thousands of individuals. In our view it is a worthwhile one.

Chapter 8

CONCLUDING OBSERVATIONS

I. THE PATIENTS

The basic facts of this investigation have been presented. Chapter 3 summarized the major questions we set out to study and the principal findings bearing on each. Chapters 5 and 6 provided more detailed data on these questions and considered the meaning of specific findings. Chapter 7 sought to approach the total experience at a different level—as an observational-impressionistic account of the human side of the investigation. In this final chapter, we propose to step back for a moment from all that we have thus far considered, without being constrained by fine points of detail. The aim in so doing is to present an overview of how empirical findings and clinical observations add up, and of how the knowledge gained from this study may modify views about several core mental health issues, which served as the motivation for our work, and were initially considered in Chapter 1.

With respect to the target patients, a simple summary is that the interventive program was to some extent helpful, but by no means comprised a basic solution to the awesome problems of chronic, entrenched schizophrenia and chronic hospitalization. However, the latter goal was entirely beyond the scope of our work. While the complexity and unevenness of our findings are not adequately reflected in the foregoing statements, there is a substantial kernel of truth in them. Although it is the dominant theme of our story, like other simplified themes it is one with many potential variations.

We have found, for example, that the particular combination of female student leaders and male patients was, by far, our most effective one—a result that simultaneously supports Poser's earlier findings and highlights a limitation of his and our work. We have also learned that initially more profoundly disturbed patients stand to gain the most from a college-student volunteer program of this type. Ironically, such a gain may reflect little more than the fact that these individuals had, through long-term hospitalization, lost their "will to fight" and no longer had strength to refuse the program or to be frightened by it. Unquestionably, student leaders felt that the patients' behavior improved significantly during the group meetings, though there is little reason to assume that these gains, if real, generalized to the ward. On several grounds, both empirical and observational, it is also clear that patients developed a fonder, more acceptant image of college students and that the program "meant something" to them.

There is evidence suggesting that program patients were significantly "better-off" than controls at the follow-up point, one year after the program had ended. Unfortunately, the term "better off" is measured here in inches, when many miles of improvement are needed to define a significantly improved life adjustment. The limitations of the program lie precisely in that observation. Less than 10% of the patients achieved a dramatically different status such as family and convalescent care or discharge to a reasonably effective community existence. Whether this failing was due to lack of outside care or patient-return facilities, or to conservative hospital discharge policies, it testifies to the fact that our program was, at best, one of limited scope when evaluated against the criterion of meaningful, stable patient discharge. To approach the latter criterion, far more sweeping, programmatic changes are needed in rehabilitation systems, in which the use of nonprofessionals would be but one aspect of a broader community-based operation.

By the preceding analysis, we wish neither to criticize our own efforts nor to engage in self-flagellation. Rather, it establishes a perspective that is helpful in thinking through where programs such as the present one belong in comprehensive future planning for chronic mental patients. The nub of the problem lies in the fact that chronic psychosis is, and will likely continue to be, irreparably debilitating, short of profound social-system change. Moreover, it renders its victims vulnerable to conditions of living, as represented by the total institution, that dehumanize him, increase his dysfunction, and encourage him to become resigned, apathetic and unwilling, or incapable, of continuing life's struggle. Programs such as ours, while perhaps well described by the terms "energizing," "mobilizing," "catalyzing," or "reawakening," remain, in the last analysis, as encapsulated oases in the otherwise stark, barren, psychologically impoverished existences of mental hospital inmates. Even their salutary effects seem to be momentary and palliative, given the adversities both of the patient's prior learning history, which contributes importantly to present pathological processes, and of his current life circumstances. The breakthrough that this program offers some patients may help them to find a new, and more meaningful adjustive plateau. For most, however, the program, unless built into a more comprehensive system-oriented treatment package, can be little more than a momentary breath of fresh air—a brief reacquaintance with positive affect and warm feeling—that precedes a return to the stark reality of their surround. If there is one clinical observation that stood out above all others, it was the dramatic, sometimes instantaneous, regression of patients to sadness and listlessness as group meetings ended and they marched back to their wards.

II. LESSONS LEARNED AND TO BE LEARNED

An important lesson learned in this study underscores the view that the soundest approach to major mental illness is to prevent its occurrence in the first place. While this goal is far easier to verbalize than to achieve, the tenacity of entrenched disorder and its dire human toll necessitates that we keep the ideal firmly in mind. The engineering of social systems and primary institutions that build psychological strengths and resources in individuals, and the development of programs for early detection of dysfunction in the organism's life history, combined with early secondary intervention, are approaches that must be followed if we are eventually to cut down the flow of major mental illness (Cowen, 1967; Zax & Cowen, 1972). The long-range answer must come from averting the onset of these conditions, since once a certain deteriorative point is reached, there is little chance for reversing its course. For established schizophrenia, reversal requires substantial change in social systems and in rehabilitative programming.

In essence, we believe that college-student volunteer programs, however useful they are, do not by themselves offer a basic solution to the problem of chronic schizophrenia. This is not to say that student volunteer programs in general, or ours in particular, are worthless. Far from it! In the present case the program clearly served some energizing or reawakening function in a number of long-dormant patients. Evidence for this is found in both objective data and clinical observations. Long-isolated, apathetic patients were able to interact with other human beings, to relate to them, and to enjoy moments of life. Even such a temporary value is not to be lightly dismissed, given their empty prior existence. For some few patients substantial gains were maintained. Though they were numerically few, the value of such gain, measured against the patient's prior long-term baseline, is considerable. Such ends certainly justify the program, while at the same time reminding us of the need for its embedding in a more comprehensive treatment package.

In the final analysis, target patients in the present program were as malfunctioning psychologically as human beings can be. Their totally chronic state is well attested to by the datum of an average of 13 years of confinement in a total institution prior to the start of the study. If we assume that the major effect of the program was to stimulate, reawaken and help patients to engage a segment of life, this value is helpful, but given the prior processes of their disorder and the current miring context of their existence, it is far from enough. The program took up only 1 or 2 hours of a 168-hour week, the rest of which was replete with vectors, both implicit and explicit, that ran counter to its aims and thrust. Conceivably, a program of this type could have more positive value for acute patients, not yet dragged down either by the long-term process effects of their own experiential history or by unfortunate living conditions. For chronic patients it, alone, is simply insufficient.

III. FUTURE PROSPECTS

While we have spoken of the theoretical need and merit of preventing major mental illness, we recognize that this is an ideal and are aware that chronic psychoses will be with us for many years to come. Is there a place for college-student volunteer programs in future approaches to such disorders? The answer to this question, while affirmative, requires elaboration, given the apparent insufficiency of student programs as isolated entities. Quite probably the most effective use of volunteer programs would be as part of a comprehensive, multifaceted attack on the problem of chronic mental disorder

Such an attack should start with settings that are engineered to promote well-being in the first place—where the institution itself does not, by its very being, tell the patient that here is a place to be sick and to give up forever. Programs that have exemplified this include those in socioenvironmental treatment (e.g., Ellsworth, 1968; Colarelli & Siegel, 1968; Sanders *et al.*, 1967) and those based on behavior modification approaches (e.g., Paul, 1969; Ayllon & Azrin, 1969). Gains will be furthered by a systematic therapeutic orientation in which goals shift from the custodial to active patient-helping ones. A therapeutic orientation is achieved not only through the activities of professionals, but also by establishing meaningful and viable helping roles—a genuine involvement in the helping enterprise—for nonprofessional personnel including, particularly, the ward attendant. Additionally, there is a need to capitalize on existing patient resources, to reduce the traditional institution-community discontinuity, and to create intermediate settings which permit the patient to move out to the community, while retaining the shelter and protection he requires (e.g., Fairweather *et al.*, 1969). Given such a multifaceted attack on chronic dysfunction, predicated on hope rather than despair, a college-student volunteer program can serve a significant catalyzing and supportive function, and can contribute to more substantial patient-growth than was achieved in the present investigation. Potential resources for such an effort, as for example, using nonprofessionals as significant others in the *community,* remain largely untapped.

IV. STUDENT VOLUNTEERS

While patients were admittedly center-stage in the present piece, they were not the only players. Certainly, the student leaders had significant roles. These individuals, not readily discriminable at the start of the program from their college-student peers, knew that they had been through a real, challenging, and different human and educational experience by the time the program ended. In the main, we made little progress in this study in identifying the so-called "effective student leader." Perhaps this was inevitable, given the homogeneity of the student group in age, prior training, orientation, and bearing. Moreover, unanticipated misfirings of design and limited patient improvement also reduced the possibility of finding correlates of leader effectiveness. Indeed, on this dimension, the high level of involvement and enthusiasm of virtually all student volunteers may have been the greatest equalizer of all.

That we failed to identify systematically correlates of effective leadership does not imply that this is a dead-end question. The likelihood of finding such correlates will increase with greater variability in volunteers and in outcomes than existed in the present study. The potential relation between attributes and attitudes of helping people, whether professionals or nonprofessionals, and the effectiveness of the service they provide for target individuals, is of considerable theoretical importance. In a situation of limited, indeed scarce, resources, that well characterizes our current mental-health helping structure, it is important to identify before-the-fact types of humans pairings that optimize the likelihood of positive outcomes in given situations.

As a result of their participation in this program, many changes occurred in the student leaders, both as individuals and as a group. Some of these changes, especially group ones, are easier to document than others, because they are based on hard data. We know, for example, that students became closely identified with patients, more acceptant of them, and more concerned about their plight. In their identification with patients, they became more alienated from the hospital as an institutional structure and, in near unilateral ways, externalized blame for the patients' unfortunate lot in the system.

There was not, in the authors' view, a single student leader who took the program as "soft duty" or as a "lark." All were deeply committed and involved to a far greater extent than in the modal college course. Though anxious, even desperate, moments were never lacking, there was always a prevailing sentiment that this program was "for real," and that the actions and involvement of students had the potential for breathing psychological life into the existence of those who had largely abandoned life's struggles. This was not a game! This was having a real stake in a real problem in a real world. As such, the program answered well the clarion call for involvement and relevance, echoing on most college campuses today.

The depth of student involvement and committment was such that the reactions they experienced—whether frustration and despair, or optimism–excitement and joy, were intense. Half-way or intellectualized responses were uncommon. This pattern of immersion can be maturing and sobering. The starkness of the hospital reality perceived by students virtually forced them to come to grips not only with inescapable issues of patient plight, but also with underlying concerns about a social system that produced such endproducts, and a setting that seemed to reinforce and perpetuate illness. Given the stage of their careers, their flexibility, and their own search for identity and direction, the experience necessarily had high impact. For more than a few, it was decisive in structuring decisions to pursue careers as professionals in mental health or closely related activities, as for example, urban planning or teaching emotionally disturbed children.

Thus there is reason to believe that the experience was more meaningful and helpful to students than to patients. The training model used in the study seems, even in retrospect, to have been an eminently sensible one. Graduate students in the program had a front-line exposure to consultation, liaison in the setting, and recruitment, training, and supervision of nonprofessionals, each a harbinger of future roles for mental health professionals. Undergraduates had meaningful clinical contact with individuals in grave psychological distress. Using this model, the reach of the helping operation underwent a much needed geometric augmentation. Thus there was simultaneous furtherance, through the program, of the mutually supportive objectives of graduate education in the mental health professions, action-oriented undergraduate education, and program development in community mental health and patient care. In this mix, the graduate student consultant stood in the same relation to undergraduate "worker-bees" as mental health professionals in the community to nonprofessional helpers.

Without question, this common pursuit of a set of clearly perceived goals and shared objectives fostered an "esprit de corps" among participants that sustained the program in its darker moments, and is cherished, in retrospect, by those who were part of it. The people involved, especially student leaders, but also the authors, worked diligently and faithfully on the task at hand. Whatever the failings of the program, they were not due to incomplete effort on anyone's part. The immediate values to students of perceived educational satisfaction, change in attitude toward mental hospital patients, and career choice, are easier to pin down than longer range, less palpable ones that pertain to their future roles as citizens and community representatives. Certainly our student leaders are better informed, more understanding of, and oriented to contemporary social problems in the area of major mental illness. Most of these gains came less from the classroom and more from their direct first-hand encounters with patients and with the institution.

V. THE SETTING

A final, quite important area for evaluation, is the effect of the program on the hospital as a setting. This is extremely difficult to assess, since our deeper concerns are with long-range, rather than momentary-reactive, effects. At the latter level, greater acceptance of the program in the hospital was evident during its course, not only in the shifting attitudes of key personnel, but also concretely through provision of materials, supplies and facilities to improve its operation. It was the hospital administrators themselves who initiated inquiry and action to continue the program for the following year. Whether this represented a change in policy or a specific gesture to people who had become known and trusted is difficult to know. If, however, the program moved hospital policy one just noticeable step away from a custodial orientation toward a more active treatment philosophy, it served a vital function, well.

VI. SUMMING UP

In bold relief, the principal lessons we have learned from this experience are the following:

(1) Gains accruing to patients, while demonstrable and real, were of the order of "baby steps" rather than "giant steps," measured against the awesome scope of their presenting problems.

(2) Initial prevention of dysfunction rather than palliation of entrenched disorder is a conceptual approach of choice for engaging the unsolved problems of major mental illness.

(3) Student volunteer programs for chronic mental patients will be most effective as they move away from being encapsulated narrow entities in a bleak surround, and become one important segment of an active, concerted, treatment-oriented approach. The latter should begin with the articulation of a facilitative setting, reduce patient isolation and

dehumanization, capitalize on existing patient resources, and end with close ties to community-based transition and after-care facilities.

(4) Program gains to participating students were considerable, whether assessed by formal research methodology, personal observation and reaction, or clinical report.

The program we have developed and described in this volume is a useful and eminently justifiable one. While it does not, nor was it intended to, stand as a comprehensive overall solution to the compelling problems of major mental illness in America today, it points to a promising direction in patient care when combined with other necessary systemic change.

REFERENCES

Albee, G. W. *Mental health manpower trends.* New York: Basic Books, 1959.

Albee, G. W. American psychology in the sixties. *American Psychologist,* 1963, **18**, 90-95.

Albee, G. W. Give us a place to stand and we will move the earth. In J. G. Harris (Ed.), *Mental health manpower needs in psychology.* Lexington, Kentucky: Univ. of Kentucky, 1966. Pp. 15-25.

Albee, G. W. The relation of conceptual models to the manpower problem. In E. L. Cowen, E. A. Gardner, & M. Zax (Eds.), *Emergent approaches to mental health problems,* New York: Appleton, 1967. Pp. 63-73. (a)

Albee, G. W. It only hurts when I laugh. *The Clinical Psychologist, Newsletter Division Twelve, American Psychological Association,* 1967, **20**, 137-139. (b)

Albee, G. W. The relation of conceptual models of disturbed behavior to institutional and manpower requirements. In F. N. Arnhoff, E. A. Rubinstein, & J. C. Speisman (Eds.), *Manpower for mental health.* Chicago: Aldine, 1969. Pp. 93-111.

Alexander, F. G., & Selesnick, S. T. *The history of psychiatry.* New York: Harper and Row, 1966.

Anker, J. M., & Walsh, R. P. Group psychotherapy, a special activity program, and a group structure in the treatment of chronic schizophrenics. *Journal of Consulting Psychology.* 1961, **25**, 476-481.

Apfelbaum, B. *Dimensions of transference in psychotherapy.* Berkeley: Univ. of California Press, 1958.

Appleby, L. Evaluation of treatment methods for chronic schizophrenics. *Archives of General Psychiatry,* 1963, **8**, 8-21.

Arieti, S. *Interpretation of schizophrenia.* New York: Robert Brunner, 1955.

Arnhoff, F. N., Rubenstein, E. A., & Speisman, J. C. (Eds.), *Manpower for mental health.* Chicago, Aldine, 1969.

Arnhoff, F. N., & Speisman, J. C. Summary and conclusions. In F. N. Arnhoff, E. A. Rubenstein, & J. C. Speisman (Eds.), *Manpower for mental health.* Chicago: Aldine, 1969. Pp. 185-197.

Ayllon, T. Intensive treatment of psychotic patients by stimulus satiation and food reinforcement. *Behavior Research and Therapy*, 1963, **1**, 53-61.

Ayllon, T., & Azrin, N. H. *The token economy.* New York: Appelton, 1969.

Babcock, H., & Levy, L. *Test and manual of direction: The revised examination for the measurement of efficiency of mental functioning.* Chicago: Stoelting, 1940.

Beck, J. C., Kantor, D., & Gelineau, V. A. Follow-up study of chronic patients "treated" by college case aide volunteers. *American Journal of Psychiatry, 1963,* **120**, 269-271.

Beers, C. W. *A mind that found itself*, 5th ed., New York: Doubleday, 1921.

Berzins, J. I., Geller, J. D., Rogers, G. W., & Rickers-Ovsiankina, M. A. Four categories for the analyses of patient-therapist role expectancies during psychotherapy. Unpublished manuscript, Univ. of Kentucky, 1966.

Berzins, J. I., & Seidman, E. Subjective reactions of A and B quasi-therapist to schizoid and neurotic communication: A replication and extension. *Journal of Consulting and Clinical Psychology*, 1968, **32**, 342-347.

Berzins, J. I., & Seidman, E. Differential therapeutic responding of A and B quasi-therapies to schizoid and neurotic communications. *Journal of Consulting and Clinical Psychology*, 1969, **33**, 279-286.

Betz, B. J. Experiences in research in psychotherapy with schizophrenic patients. In H. H. Strupp & L. Luborsky (Eds.), *Research in psychotherapy*, Vol. 2. Washington, D. C.: American Psychological Association, 1962. Pp. 41-60.

Betz, B. J. The problem solving approach and therapeutic effectiveness. *American Journal of Psychotherapy*, 1966, **20**, 45-56.

Bockhoven, J. S. *Moral treatment in American psychiatry.* New York: Springer, 1963.

Braginsky, B. M., Braginsky, D. D., & Ring, K. *Methods of madness: The mental hospital as a last resort.* New York: Holt, 1969.

Buss, A. H., & Lang, P. J. Psychological deficit in schizophrenia: Affect, reinforcement, and concept attainment. *Journal of Abnormal Psychology*, 1965, **70**, 74-90.

Carkhuff, R. R. *Helping and human relations: A primer for lay and professional helpers. Vol. I Selection and training.* New York: Holt, 1969. (a)

Carkhuff, R. R. *Helping and human relations: A primer for lay and professional helpers. Vol. II Practice and Research.* New York: Holt, 1969. (b)

Carkhuff, R. R., & Truax, C. B. Lay mental health counseling: The effects of lay group counseling, *Journal of Consulting Psychology*, 1965, **29**, 426-431.

Carson, R. C., Harden, J. A., & Shows, W. D. The A-B distinction and behavior in quasi-therapeutic situations. *Journal of Consulting Psychology*, 1964, **28**, 426-433.

Chapin, F. S. Preliminary standardization of a social insight scale. *American Sociological Review*, 1942, **7**, 211-225.

Chapman, L., Chapman, J. P., & Miller, G. A. A theory of verbal behavior in schizophrenia. In B. Maher (Ed.), *Progress in experimental personality research.* Vol. 2, New York: Academic Press, 1964. Pp. 46-79.

Chinsky, J. M. Nonprofessionals in a mental hospital: A study of the college student volunteer. (Unpublished doctoral dissertation.) Univ. of Rochester, 1968.

Chinsky, J. M., & Rappaport, J. Attitude change among college students and chronic patients: A dual perspective. *Journal of Consulting and Clinical Psychology*, 1970, **35**, 388-394.

Chinsky, J. M., & Rappaport, J. Evaluation of a technique for the behavioral assessment of nonprofessionals. *Journal of Clinical Psychology*, 1971, **27**, 400-402.

Chinsky, J. M., & Rappaport, J. Brief critique of the meaning and reliability of "Accurate Empathy" ratings. *Psychological Bulletin*, 1970, **73**, 379-382.

Colarelli, N. J., & Siegel, S. M. Administrative structure and treatment goals: Diprhythmia? *Mental Hospitals*, 1963, **14**, 608-612.

Colarelli, N. J., & Siegel, S. M. *Ward H: An adventure in innovation.* Princeton, New Jersey: Van Nostrand, 1966.

Colby, K. M. Psychotherapeutic process. *Annual Review of Psychology,* 1964, **15**, 347-370.

Cowen, E. L. Overview and directions for future work. In E. L. Cowen, E. A. Gardner, & M. Zax (Eds.), *Emergent approaches to mental health problems.* New York: Appleton, 1967. Pp. 389-455.

Cowen, E. L., Carlisle, R., & Kaufman, G. Evaluation of a college student volunteers program with primary graders experiencing school adjustment problems. *Psychology in the Schools,* 1969, **6**, 371-375.

Cowen, E. L., Chinsky, J. M., & Rappaport, J. An undergraduate practicum in community mental health. *Community Mental Health Journal,* 1970, **6**, 91-100.

Cowen, E. L., Gardner, E. A., & Zax, M. *Emergent approaches to mental health problems.* New York: Appleton, 1967.

Cowen, E. L., & Zax, M., The mental health fields today: Issues and problems. In E. L. Cowen, E. A. Gardner, & M. Zax (Eds.) *Emergent approaches to mental health problems.* New York: Appleton, 1967. Pp. 3-29.

Cowen, E. L., Zax, M., & Laird, J. D. A college student volunteer program in an elementary school setting. *Community Mental Health Journal,* 1966, **2**, 319-328.

Cumming, E., & Henry, W. E. *Growing old.* New York: Basic Books, 1961.

Davison, G. C. Appraisal of behavior modification techniques with adults in institutional settings. In C. M. Franks (Ed.). *Assessment and status of the behavioral therapies and associated developments.* New York: McGraw-Hill, 1969.

Dunn, L. M. *Expanded manual for the Peabody Picture Vocabulary Test.* Beverly Hills, California: Western Psychological Services, 1959.

Edwards, A. L. Social desirability and description of others. *Journal of Abnormal and Social Psychology,* 1959, **59**, 434-436.

Ellsworth, R. B. *The M.A.C.C. Behavioral Adjustment Scale* (Form II). Beverly Hills, California: Western Psychological Services, 1962.

Ellsworth, R. B. *Non-professionals in psychiatric rehabilitation.* New York: Appleton, 1968.

Eysenck, H. J. *The scientific study of personality.* London: Routledge and Kegan Paul, 1952.

Ewalt, P. L. *Mental health volunteers.* Springfield, Illinois: Thomas, 1967.

Fairweather, G. W. (Ed.) *Social psychology in treating mental illness: An experimental approach.* New York: Wiley, 1964.

Fairweather, G. W. *Methods for experimental social innovation.* New York: Wiley, 1967.

Fairweather, G. W., Sanders, P. H., Cressler, D. L., & Maynard, H. *Community life for the mentally ill. An alternative to institutional care.* Chicago: Aldine, 1969.

Felix, R. H. *Mental illness: Progress and prospects.* New York: Columbia Univ. Press, 1967.

Foucoult, M. *Madness and civilization: A history of insanity in the age of reason.* New York: Mentor, 1965.

Gendlin, E. T. Research in psychotherapy with schizophrenic patients and the nature of that "illness." *American Journal of Psychotherapy.* 1966, **20**, 4-16.

Goffman, E. *Asylums.* Garden City, New York: Doubleday, 1961.

Goldstein, A. P. Psychotherapy research by extrapolation from social psychology, *Journal of Counseling Psychology,* 1966, **13**, 38-45.

Goodman, G. *Studying helping relationships between college students and troubled boys.* Paper presented at the meeting of the American Psychological Association, Sept. 1965.

Goodman, G. An experiment with companionship therapy: College students and troubled boys—assumptions, selection, and design. In B. G. Guerney (Ed.) *Psychotherapeutic agents: New roles for non-professionals, parents and teachers.* New York: Holt, 1969. Pp. 121-128.

Gough, H. C., & Heilbrun, A. B. *The adjective check list manual.* Palo Alto, California: Counseling Psychological Press, 1965.

Granger, G. W. Abnormalities of sensory perception. In H. J. Eysenck (Ed.) *Handbook of Abnormal Psychology.* New York: Basic Books, 1961.

Graziano, A. M. Clinical innovations and the mental health power structure: A social case history. *American Psychologist,* 1969, **24**, 10-18.

Greenblatt, M., & Kantor, D. Students and the manpower shortage. *American Journal of Psychiatry,* 1962, **118**, 809-814.

Greenblatt, M., & Levinson, D. J. Mental hospitals. In B. Wolman (Ed.) *Handbook of Clinical Psychology.* New York: McGraw-Hill, 1965. Pp. 1343-1359.

Grob, G. N. The state mental hospital in mid-nineteenth century America: A social analysis. *American Psychologist,* 1966, **21**, 510-523.

Grosser, C., Henry, W. E., & Kelly, J. G. (Eds.). *Non-professionals in the human services.* San Francisco: Jossey-Bass, 1969.

Guerney, B. G. (Ed.). *Psychotherapeutic agents: New roles for non-professional parents, and teachers.* New York: Holt, 1969.

Harrington, M. *The other America: Poverty in the United States.* New York: Penguin, 1962.

Harris, J. G. (Ed.). *Mental health manpower needs in psychology.* Lexington, Kentucky: Univ. of Kentucky, 1966.

Hays, W. *Statistics for psychologists.* New York: Holt, 1966.

Holzberg, J. D. The companion program: Implementing the manpower recommendations of the Joint Commission on Mental Illness and Health. *American Psychologist,* 1963, **18**, 224-226.

Holzberg, J. D., & Gewirtz, H. Changes in self-acceptance and moral judgement in college students as a function of companionship with hospitalized mental patients. *Journal of Consulting Psychology,* 1964, **28**, 299-303.

Holzberg, J. D., Gewirtz, H., & Ebner, E. Changes in moral judgement and self acceptance as a function of companionship with hospitalized mental patients *Journal of Consulting Psychology,* 1964, **28**, 299-303.

Holzberg, J. D., & Knapp, R. H. The social interaction of college students and chronically ill mental patients. *American Journal of Orthopsychiatry,* 1965, **35**, 487-492.

Holzberg, J. D., Knapp, R. H., & Turner, J. L. Companionship with the mentally ill: Effects on the personalities of college student volunteers. *Psychiatry,* 1966, **29**, 395-405.

Holzberg, J. D., Knapp, R. H., & Turner, J. L. College students as companions to the mentally ill. In E. L. Cowen, E. A. Gardner, & M. Zax (Eds.) *Emergent approaches to mental health problems.* New York: Appleton, 1967. Pp. 91-109.

Holzberg, J. D., Whiting, H. S., & Lowy, D. G. Chronic patients and a college companion program. *Mental Hospital,* 1964, **15**, 152-158.

Jackson, D. M. The development and evaluation of the personality research form. Unpublished manuscript, Univ. of Ontario, 1965.

Jensen, A. Scoring the Stroop test. *Acta Psychologica,* 1965, **24**, 398-408.

Jensen, A., & Rohwer, W. D. The Stroop color word test: A reveiw. *Acta Psychologica,* 1966, **25**, 63-93.

Joint Commission on Mental Illness and Health. *Action for mental health.* New York: Basic Books, 1961.

Jones, M. *The therapeutic community.* New York: Basic Books, 1953.

Jones, M. *Beyond the therapeutic community.* New Haven, Connecticut: Yale Univ. Press, 1968.

Jourard, S. M. *The transparent self.* Princeton, New Jersey: Van Nostrand, 1964.

Kandel, D. B., & Williams, R. H. *Psychiatric rehabilitation: Some problems of research.* New York: Atherton, 1964.

Kemp, D. E. Correlates of the Whitehorn-Betz A–B scale in a quasi-therapeutic situation. *Journal of Consulting Psychology,* 1966, **30,** 509-516.

Kety, S. S. The relevance of biochemical studies to the etiology of schizophrenia. In J. R. Romano (Ed.) *The origins of schizophrenia.* Amsterdam: Excerpta Medica, 1967. Pp. 35-41.

Kiesler, D. J. Some myths of psychotherapy research and the search for a paradigm. *Psychological Bulletin,* 1966, **65,** 110-136.

Klein, W. L., & Zax, M. The use of a hospital volunteer program in the teaching of abnormal psychology. *Journal of Social Psychology,* 1965, **65,** 155-165.

Knapp, R. H., & Holzberg, J. D. Characteristics of college students volunteering for service to mental patients. *Journal of Consulting Psychology,* 1964, **28,** 82-85.

Lang, P. J., & Buss, A. H. Psychological deficit in schizophrenia: II. Interference and activation. *Journal of Abnormal Psychology,* 1965, **70,** 77-106.

Lorr, M., & McNair, D. M. Evidence of ten psychotic syndromes. *Journal of Consulting Psychology,* 1962, **26,** 185-189.

Lorr, M., & McNair, D. M. Methods relating to evaluation of therapeutic outcomes. In L. A. Gottschalk & A. H. Auerbach (Eds.) *Methods of research in psychotherapy.* New York: Appleton, 1966.

Luborsky, L., & Strupp, H. H. Research problems in psychotherapy: A three-year follow-up. In H. H. Strupp & L. Luborsky (Eds.) *Research in psychotherapy,* Vol. II. Washington, D.C.: American Psychological Association, 1962. Pp. 308-329.

Lyerly, S. B., & Abbott, P. S. *Handbook of psychiatric rating scales* (1950-1964). Public Health Service Publications No. 1495, 1966, National Institute of Mental Health.

Mace, D. L. College volunteers as group leaders with chronic patients: Effects of ward personnel involvement on ward behavior change. (Unpublished doctoral dissertation.) Univ. of Rochester, 1969.

Maher, B. A., *Principles of psychopathology.* New York: McGraw-Hill, 1966.

McNemar, Q. *Psychological statistics,* 3rd ed. New York: Wiley, 1962.

Mendel, W. M. & Rapport, S. Outpatient treatment for chronic schizophrenic patients: Therapeutic consequences of an existential view. *Archives of General Psychiatry,* 1963, **8,** 190-196.

Mischel, W. *Personality and assessment.* New York: Wiley, 1968.

Mischel, W. Continuity and change in personality. *American Psychologist,* 1969, **24,** 1012-1018.

Mogar, R. E. Research in psychedelic drug therapy: A critical analysis. In J. M. Schlein (Ed.), *Research in psychotherapy,* Vol. III. Washington, D. C.: American Psychological Association, 1968. Pp. 500-511.

Murray, H. A., *Explorations in personality.* New York: Oxford, 1935.

National Institutes of Mental Health. Student volunteers at state mental hospitals. *Mental Health News Digest,* 1968, 28-29.

Noyes, A. P., & Kolb, L. C. *Modern clinical psychiatry.* Philadelphia: Sanders, 1958.

O'Connor, R. D., & Rappaport, J. Application of social learning principles to the training of ghetto blacks. *American Psychologist,* 1970, **25,** 659-661.

Osgood, C. E., Suci, G. J., & Tannenbaum, P. H. *The measurement of meaning.* Urbana, Illinois: Univ. of Illinois Press, 1957.

Parloff, M. B., Kelman, H. C., & Frank, J. D. Comfort, effectiveness, and self-awareness as criteria of improvement in psychotherapy. *American Journal of Psychiatry* 1954, **111,** 343-351.

Paul, G. L. Chronic mental patient: Current status—future directions. *Psychological Bulletin,* 1969, **71**, 81-94.

Payne, R. W., Ancevich, S. S., & Laverty, S. B. Overinclusive thinking in symptom-free schizophrenics. *Canadian Psychiatric Association Journal,* 1963, **8**, 225-234.

Payne, R. W., & Caird, W. K. Reaction time, distractability, and overinclusive thinking in psychotics. *Journal of Abnormal Psychology,* 1967, **72**, 112-121.

Poser, E. G. The effect of therapist training on group therapeutic outcome. *Journal of Consulting Psychology,* 1966, **30**, 283-289.

Rappaport, J. Nonprofessionals in a mental hospital: College students as group leaders with chronic patients. (Unpublished doctoral dissertation.) Univ. of Rochester, 1968.

Rappaport, J., & Chinsky, J. M. Nonprofessionals as mental health workers in a state hospital setting: A preliminary report. Paper presented at annual meeting of the Eastern Psychological Association, Washington, D.C., April, 1968.

Rappaport, J., & Chinsky, J. M. Behavior ratings of chronic patients: Cross-situational and cross-rater agreement. *Journal of Consulting and Clinical Psychology,* 1970, **34**, 394-397.

Rappaport, J., & Chinsky, J. M. "Accurate Empathy": Confusion of Construct. *Psychological Bulletin,* 1971, **70**, in press.

Rappaport, J., & O'Connor, R. D. The psychological center in a psychology department. In B. Saper (Ed.) The campus institute or center. Symposium presented at the convention of the Amercian Psychological Association, Miami, 1970.

Raush, H. L., & Raush, C. L. *The half-way house movement: A search for sanity.* New York: Appleton, 1968.

Reiff, R. Mental health manpower and institutional change. In E. L. Cowen, E. A. Gardner, & M. Zax (Eds.) *Emergent approaches to mental health problems.* New York: Appleton, 1967. Pp. 74-88.

Reiff, R., & Riessman, F. The indigenous nonprofessional: A strategy of change in community action and community mental health programs. *Community Mental Health Journal,* Monograph No. 1, 1965.

Riessman, F., Cohen, J., & Pearl, A. *Mental health of the poor.* New York: Free Press, 1964.

Rioch, M. J. Changing concepts in the training of therapists. *Journal of Consulting Psychology,* 1966, **30**, 290-292.

Rioch, M. J. Pilot projects in training mental health counselors. In E. L. Cowen, E. A. Gardner, & M. Zax (Eds.) *Emergent approaches to mental health problems.* New York: Appleton, 1967. Pp. 110-127.

Romano, J. R. (Ed.) *The origins of schizophrenia.* Amsterdam: Excerpta Medica, 1967.

Rosenbaum, M. Some comments on the use of untrained therapists. *Journal of Consulting Psychology,* 1966, **30**, 292-294.

Rotter, J. B. *Social learning and clinical psychology.* Englewood Cliffs, New Jersey: Prentice Hall, 1954.

Rotter, J. B. Generalized expantancies for internal versus external control of reinforcement. *Psychological Monographs,* 1966, **80** (Whole No. 609).

Rubenstein, R., & Lasswell, H. D. *The sharing of power in a psychiatric hospital.* New Haven, Connecticut: Yale Univ. Press, 1966.

Rundquist, E. A. Item and response characteristics in attitude and personality measurement: A reaction to L. G. Rorer's "The great response style myth." *Psychological Bulletin,* 1966, **66**, 166-177.

Sanders, R. New manpower for mental hospital service. In E. L. Cowen, E. A. Gardner, & M. Zax (Eds.) *Emergent approaches to mental health problems.* New York: Appleton, 1967. Pp. 128-143.

Sanders, R., Smith, R. S., & Weinman, B. S. *Chronic psychoses and recovery: An experiment in socio-environmental treatment.* San Francisco: Jossey-Bass, 1967.

Sarason, I. G., & Ganzer, V. J. Social influence techniques in clinical and community psychology. In C. D. Spielberger (Ed.) *Current topics in clinical and community psychology,* Vol. I. New York: Academic Press, 1969. Pp. 1-66;

Scheff, T. J. *Being mentally ill: A sociological theory.* Chicago: Aldine, 1966.

Scheibe, K. E. College students spend eight weeks in a mental hospital: A case report. *Psychotherapy: Theory, Research, and Practice,* 1965, 2, 117-120.

Scheibe, K. E., Kulik, J. A., Hersch, P. D., & La Macchia, S. College students on chronic wards. *Community Mental Health Journal,* Monograph Series, No. 5, 1969, 33 pp.

Schofield, W. *Psychotherapy: The purchase of friendship.* Englewood Cliffs, New Jersey: Prentice-Hall, 1964.

Schooler, C. Affiliation among schizophrenics: Preferred characteristics of the other. *Journal of Nervous and Mental Diseases,* 1963, **37**, 438-446.

Selling, L. S. *Men against madness.* New York: Greenberg, 1940.

Shakow, D. Segmental set: A theory of the formal psychological deficit in schizophrenia, *Archives of General Psychiatry,* 1962, **6**, 1-17.

Shows, W. D., & Carson, R. C. The A-B therapist "type" distinction and spatial orientation: Replication and extension. *Journal of Nervous and Mental Diseases,* 1965, **141**, 456-462.

Siegel, S. *Nonparametric statistics for the behavioral sciences,* New York: McGraw, 1956.

Sobey, F. *The nonprofessional revolution in mental health.* New York: Columbia Univ. Press, 1970.

Steer, H. O., & Allen, M. E. *Cerebral palsey research project.* Ontario, Canada: Ontario Society for Crippled Children, 1960.

Thurstone, L. L., & Mellinger, J. J. *The Stroop test,* The psychometric laboratory, Univ. of North Carolina, 1953.

Tourney, G., Bloom, V., Lowenger, P. L., Schorer, C., Auld, F., & Grisell, J. A study of psychotherapeutic process variables in psychoneurotic and schizophrenic patients. *American Journal of Psychotherapy,* 1966, **20**, 112-124.

Truax, C. B. The process of group psychotherapy relationships between hypothesized therapeutic conditions and interpersonal exploration. *Psychological Monographs,* 1961, **75** (Whole no. 511).

Truax, C. B. Reinforcement and non-reinforcement in Rogerian psychotherapy. *Journal of Abnormal Psychology,* 1966, **71**, 1-9.

Truax, C. B., & Carkhuff, R. R. *Toward effective counseling and psychotherapy: Training and practice.* Chicago: Aldine, 1967.

Turner, J. L., Holzberg, J. D., & Knapp, R. H. Effects of companionship with mental patients on students' stereotypes of the typical mental patient. Paper presented at the meeting of the Eastern Psychological Association, Boston, April, 1967.

Ullmann, L. P. *Institution and outcome: A comparative study of psychiatric hospitals.* London: Pergamon, 1967.

Umbarger, C. C., Dalsimer, J. S., Morrison, A. P., & Breggin, P. R. *College students in a mental hospital.* New York: Grune and Stratton, 1962.

Venables, P. H. Input dysfunction in schizophrenia. In B. A. Maher (Ed.), *Progress in experimental personality research,* Vol. 1. New York: Academic Press, 1964. Pp. 1-48.

Wechsler, D. *Manual for Wechsler adult intelligence scale.* New York: The Psychological Corporation, 1955.

Weckowicz, T. E. Perception of hidden pictures by schizophrenic patients. *Archives of General Psychiatry,* 1960, **2,** 521-527.

Weckowicz, T. E., & Blewett, D. B. Size constancy and abstract thinking in schizophrenia. *Journal of Mental Science,* 1959, **105,** 409-934.

Weiner, I. B. *Psychodiagnosis in schizophrenia.* New York: Wiley, 1966.

Whitehorn, J. C., & Betz, B. J. A study of psychotherapeutic relationships between physicians and schizophrenic patients. *American Journal of Psychiatry,* 1954, **111,** 321-331.

Winer, B. J. *Statistical principles in experimental design.* New York: McGraw-Hill, 1962.

Wrightsmann, L. S., Measurement of philosophies of human nature. *Psychological Reports,* 1964, **14,** 743-751.

Yates, A. J. Abnormalities of psychomotor functions. In H. J. Eysenck (Ed.) *Handbook of abnormal psychology.* New York: Basic Books, 1961. pp. 32-61.

Zax, M., & Cowen, E. L. *Abnormal psychology: Changing conceptions.* New York: Holt, 1972.

Zax, M., & Klein, A. Measurement of personality and behavior changes following psychotherapy. *Psychological Bulletin,* 1960, **57,** 435-448.

Zigler, E., & Phillips, L. Social effectiveness and symptomatic behaviors. *Journal of Abnormal and Social Psychology,* 1960, **61,** 231-238.

Zigler, E., & Phillips, L. Case history data and psychiatric diagnosis. *Journal of Consulting Psychology,* 1961, **25,** 458-465. (a)

Zigler, E., & Phillips, L. Psychiatric diagnosis: A critique. *Journal of Abnormal and Social Psychology,* 1961, **63,** 607-618. (b)

Zigler, E., & Phillips, L. Social competence and outcome in psychiatric disorder. *Journal of Abnormal and Social Psychology,* 1961, **63,** 264-271. (c)

Zilboorg, G., & Henry, G. W. *A history of medical psychology.* New York: Norton, 1941.

INDEX

A

A—B status, 29, 30, 81, 117
Accurate empathy, 29, 81, 116
 correlation with other measures, 116
  with outcome, 116-117
 reliability, 116
Adjective checklist, 32, 82, 122, 126, 128, 128, 129
After-care programs, 7-8
 half-way house, 8
Albee, G. W., 9, 11, 38, 51, 54, 55
Alexander, F. G., 3
Allen, M. E., 69
Ancevich, S. S., 68
Anker, J. M., 17, 96
Apfelbaum, B., 71, 73, 108
Appleby, L., 17
Arieti, S., 3
Arnoff, F. N., 9, 10, 12
Attitudes
 initial patient, 59, 71-73, 106, 149
 initial student, 60, 78-80, 82, 120, 122, 128, 140-142, 145-147
 patient change in, 106-110
 student change in, 32, 33, 128-133
Auld, F., 30
Ayllon, T., 7, 185
Azrin, N. H., 7, 185

B

Babcock, H., 68
Beck, J. C., 13
Beers, C., 4, 38
Behavior ratings, 69, 71, 93-96
 Ellsworth MACC behavioral adjustment scale form II, 69
 group behavior, 71, 93
 by students, 94-96
 by ward attendants, 69, 94
Berzins, J. I., 30, 71
Betz, B. J., 29, 30, 81, 117
Blewett, D. B., 69
Bloom, V., 30
Bockhoven, J. S., 37
Braginsky, B. M., 2-4, 22
Braginsky, D. D., 2-4, 22
Breggen, P. R., 12, 55
Buss, A. H., 68

C

Caird, W. K., 68
Caplan, G., 54, 55
Carkhuff, R., 17, 29, 80, 81, 83, 84, 116, 124, 134
Carlisle, R., 51

Carson, R. C., 30
Chapin, F. S., 82, 122, 126
Chapman, J. P., 68
Chapman, L., 68
Chinsky, J. M., 23, 25, 43, 45, 81, 94, 111, 116-118, 120, 122, 126 128, 134, 135
Cohen, F., 51
Colarelli, N. J., 4, 6, 17, 18, 26, 185
Colby, K. M., 28
Connecticut Valley Hospital Program, 13-14
Cowen, E. L., 1-3, 5, 9, 10, 12, 16, 23, 25, 32, 43, 49, 51, 54-56, 58, 108, 132, 184
Cressler, D. L., 8
Cumming, E., 101

D

Dalsimer, J. S., 12, 55
Davison, G. C., 7
Dix, D. L., 4, 38
Dunn, L. M., 65

E

Ebner, E., 33
Edwards, A. L., 131
Edwards Personal Preference Scale, 31
Ellsworth, R. B., 6, 18-20, 26, 42, 69, 96 101, 106, 112, 148, 185
Eysenck, H. J., 54, 55, 68

F

Fairweather, G. W., 6, 8, 21, 22, 65, 88, 90, 169, 185
Fairweather Project, 21-22
Felix, R. H., 6
Follow-up interview, 171-181
Follow-up study, 110-111
Fort Meade Project, 18-19
Foucoult, M., 4
Frank, J. D., 68

G

Gans, H., 54, 55
Ganzer, V. J., 11
Gardner, E. A., 51, 54
Gelineau, V. A., 13
Geller, J. D., 71
Gendlin, E. T., 39
Genuineness, 29, 81, 116
Gewirtz, H., 13, 33
Goffman, E., 4, 33, 40, 51, 54, 111
Goldenberg, I., 55
Goldstein, A., 71
Goodman, G., 29, 31, 81, 118
Gough, H., 32, 82
Granger, G. W., 68
Graziano, A. M., 41
Greenblatt, M., 4, 6, 13, 38, 54, 55
Grisell, J., 30
Grobb, G. N., 38
Grosser, C., 10
GroupActivities Form(GAF), 74, 87, 133, 134, 170
Group Assessment of Interpersonal Traits, (GAIT), 31, 81, 83, 84, 116-118, 120, 124, 126, 134, 139
  correlation with outcome, 118-120
Group process
  change and, 133-134
  measure, 134-137
  meeting rooms, 142-143
  meeting schedule, 143-144
  outcome and, 135
  volunteer attributes and, 134-135
Guerney, B. G., 10, 11, 73, 110

H

Haggstrom, W. C., 55, 56
Harden, J. A., 30
Harrington, M., 51, 55
Harris, J. G., 10
Harvard-Radcliffe Program, 12-13
Hays, W., 96
Heilbrun, A. B., 82
Henry, W. E., 10, 101
Hersch, P. D., 14
Holzberg, J. D., 13, 23, 31, 32, 33, 109, 126, 128, 140

I

Internal-external locus of control, 82

J

Jackson, D. N., 82
Jensen, A., 69
Joint Commission on Mental Illness and Health, ix, 2, 4-7, 38, 55
Jones, M., 6, 37
Jourard, S. M., 82, 126

K

Kandel, D. B., 26, 65
Kantor, D., 13
Kaufman, G., 51
Kelly, J. G., 10
Kelman, H. C., 68
Kemp, D. E., 30
Kety, S. S., 3
Kiesler, D. J., 28
Klein, W. L., 49, 68
Knapp, R. H., 13, 31, 32, 109, 126, 128
Kolb, L. C., 109
Kulik, J. A., 14

L

Laird, J. D., 32, 49, 132
LaMacchia, S., 14
Lang, P. J., 68
Lasswell, H. D., 4, 6, 21, 22
Laverty, S. B., 68
Levine, M., 55
Levinson, D. J., 4, 6, 38, 54, 55
Levy, L., 68
Lorr, M., 30
Lowenger, P. L., 30
Lowy, D. G., 13
Luborsky, L., 93, 106

M

Mace, D. L., 112, 113, 148
McNair, D. M., 30
McNemar, Q., 117
Maher, B. A., 68
Male patient-female volunteer combination, 93, 97-102
    characteristics and change scores, 98-100
    outcome summary, 100-102
Manpower, 9-22
    mental hospital and, 12
    new utilizations, 12-22
    shortage of, 9
Mellinger, J. J., 69
Mendel, W. M., 17
Mental hospitals, 4-9
    day hospitals, 7
    description of, 6
    effects of, 4
    improving effectiveness, 5-7
    manpower and, 12
    night hospitals, 7
Metropolitan State Hospital, 12-13
Miller, G. A., 68
Mischel, W., 95
Mogar, R. E., 93
MMPI, 32
Moral treatment, 37
Morrison, A. P., 12, 55
Murray, H. A., 82

N

Nonpossessive warmth, 29, 81, 116
Nonprofessionals, 10-35, 186-189
    attitudes of, 32
    effectiveness of, 22-28
    limits of, 27, 28
    as mental health workers, 11
    other than college students, 17
    personality attributes of, 28
    qualities of, 28
    redeployment of, 25-26
    training of, 11
Noyes, A. P., 109

O

O'Connor, R. D., 2, 11
Osgood, C. E., 82
Outcome evaluation, 91-102
    behavior ratings, 93-96
    performance measures, 91-93
Outcome measures, 68-71
    Figure-Ground Confusion Test, 69

group behavior, 71
reaction time I, 68
reaction time II, 68
Stroop Color Naming Test, 69
tapping speed, 68
verbal fluency, 69
WAIS Digit Symbol Test, 69
ward behavior, 69, 71

P

Parloff, M. B., 68
Patient-group change
average percentage improvement, 116
mean improvement method, 115
Patient outcome 91-106
behavior ratings, 93-96
demographics and, 102-106
performance measures, 91-93
premeasures and, 87-91
student personality and, 114-126
Patients, 64-73, 149, 182-184
assignment to groups, 65
attendance, 85-86, 115
attenders and nonattenders, 85
demographics and change scores, 102-106
demographic characteristics, 66-67
evaluation and, 68
follow-up, 110-111
perception of college student volunteers, 71, 106-110
sample 65-67
Patients Expectations and Perceptions Scale (PEP), 72-74, 106-111
cluster scores, 71-73, 108-110
item analysis, 106-107
Paul, G. L., 3, 6, 7, 185
Payne, R. W., 68
Pearl, A., 51
Perception of college students, 107-110
Personality Research Form (PRF) 82,122,126
Philadelphia State Hospital Project, 20-21
Philipps, L., 65, 103, 113
Philosophies of Human Nature, 82, 120, 122
Pilot project, 45-49
hospital attitudes, 46
student attitude, 45
value of, 47
Pinel, H., 4
Poser, E. G., 14-16, 23, 55, 56, 78, 96, 101, 102, 183
Pretest data, 87-91
change scores and, 102-106
Prevention, 9, 27, 184
Psychological disorder, 1-9
biochemical factors, 3
functional psychoses, 2, 8
history of, 1-3
schizophrenia, 3, 8, 30
treatment approaches, 1-9, 38, 185
Psychology Practicum Seminar, 49-55, 278
design of the course, 51
recruiting students for, 50, 52-53.

R

Rappaport, J., 2, 7, 11, 23, 25, 43, 45, 81, 89, 94, 98-100, 106, 111
Rapport, S., 17
Rausch, C. L., 8
Rausch, H. L., 8
Reiff, R., 11, 25
Research, 57-63
design, 57-59
questions, 111
summary, 61-63, 100-102, 113, 182-184, 186-189
Rickers-Ovsiankina, M. A., 71
Riessman, F., 25, 51
Ring, K., 2, 3, 4, 22
Rioch, M. J., 11, 23, 25, 55, 56, 108
Rochester State Hospital, 39-55, 140-143
Rogers, G. W., 71
Romano, J. R., 2, 3
Rosenbaum, 15, 55, 56
Rosenzweig, S., 55
Rotter, J. B., 82, 96
Rubenstein, R., 4, 6, 21, 22
Rundquist, E. A., 131

S

Sanders, D. H., 8
Sanders, R., 6, 8, 20, 21, 42, 101, 106, 185
Sanford, N., 55

Sarason, I. G., 11, 55
Scheff, T. J., 3, 4, 27
Scheibe, K. E., 14, 33, 109, 132
Schofield, W., 38, 51, 55
Schooler, C., 101
Schorer, C., 30
Seidman, E., 30
Selesnick, S. T., 3
Sarason, I. G., 11, 55
Scheff, T. J., 3, 4, 27
Scheibe, K. E., 14, 33, 109, 132
Schofield, W., 38, 51, 55
Self-disclosure inventory, 82, 120, 122
Selling, L. S., 3
Semantic differential, 82-83, 128
Shakow, D., 91, 93
Shows, W. D., 30
Siegel, S. M., 4, 6, 17, 18, 26, 106, 185
Smith, R. S., 6, 20, 42, 101
Sobey, F., 10
"Social Deepfreeze," 26
Social distance hypothesis, 25, 73
Social competence, 113
Social insight test, 82, 120, 122
Social system change, 40-44, 188
Socioenvironmental therapy, 20, 185
Spiesman, J. C., 9, 12
Steer, H. O., 69
Strupp, H. H., 93, 106
Student diaries, 145-147, 151-154, 158-167
Student outcome, 114-126
    attitude change, 128-133
    personality and, 114-116
Student volunteers, 78-84, 186-188
    attitude
        toward mental hospitals, 145-147
        patient change and, 122-126
        toward patients, 128-133, 151-154
    contrasted with nonvolunteers, 126
    control group, 79-80
    effectiveness of, 114-116
    evaluation measures, 80-84
    factor analysis of personality
        measures, 120-123
    halo effect, 95
    group process and, 134-135
    male-female differences, 126
    personality, 78, 79, 82-84, 114-126
    personality and patient change, 122-126
    reactions to project, 145-147
    recruitment, 50-51
    sample characteristics, 78-79
    "special" group, 166-167
    supervisory meetings, 75
Succi, G. J., 82

T

Tannenbaum, P. H., 82
Termination, 167-169
"Therapeutic community," 6-7, 37
Therapeutic talent, 80-81, 120
Thurstone, L. L., 69
Token economy, 7
Topeka State Hospital, 17
Tourney, G., 30
Truax, C. B., 17, 29, 80, 81, 83, 84, 116, 124, 134
Turner, J. R., 13, 32, 109, 132

U

Ullmann, L. P., 6, 12
Umbarger, C. C., 12, 55, 56
Undergraduates, 49
University of Rochester, 49, 50, 165
    Psychology 278 (Seminar-practicum), 49-55, 278

V

Venables, P. H., 68

W

Walsh, R. P., 17, 96
Ward, H Project, 17
Wechsler, D., 69
Weckowicz, T. E., 69
Weiner, I. B., 68
Weinman, B. S., 6, 20, 42, 101
Whitehorn, J. C., 29, 30, 81
Whiting, H. S., 13

Williams, R. H., 26, 65
Winer, B. J., 91, 128, 129, 134
Wolpe, J., 55, 56
Wrightsmann, L. S., 82, 122

Y

Yates, A. J., 68

Z

Zax, M., 1, 2, 3, 5, 9, 10, 12, 32, 49, 51, 54, 68, 132, 184
Zigler, E., 65, 103, 113
Zilboorg, G., 3